My ADHD Life

Life through the Eyes of a 5th Grade Girl

MG and Gram

ISBN: 9798321137581
Imprint: Independently published

Table of Contents

A Message from MG and Gram

This is the story of a 5th-grade girl named MG. MG is me, and my partner is my Gram. I have a lot to say, but I don't always know how to say it, and my Gram helps me. I have a lot of feelings. Feelings of an average ten-year-old and feelings of a ten-year-old with lots of learning problems.

The one thing I know is that my Gram loves me and cherishes me…even when I drive her crazy. I have Attention Deficit Hyperactive Disorder (ADHD.) Many people say this makes me creative, curious, and energetic. It also makes me struggle, feel sad, and want just to be a normal kid.

ADHD can be a tricky companion to navigate life with, but, I am learning all the time. Some days I think I will conquer it, and some days I think it will conquer me.

My ever-supportive Gram provides wisdom and insight,

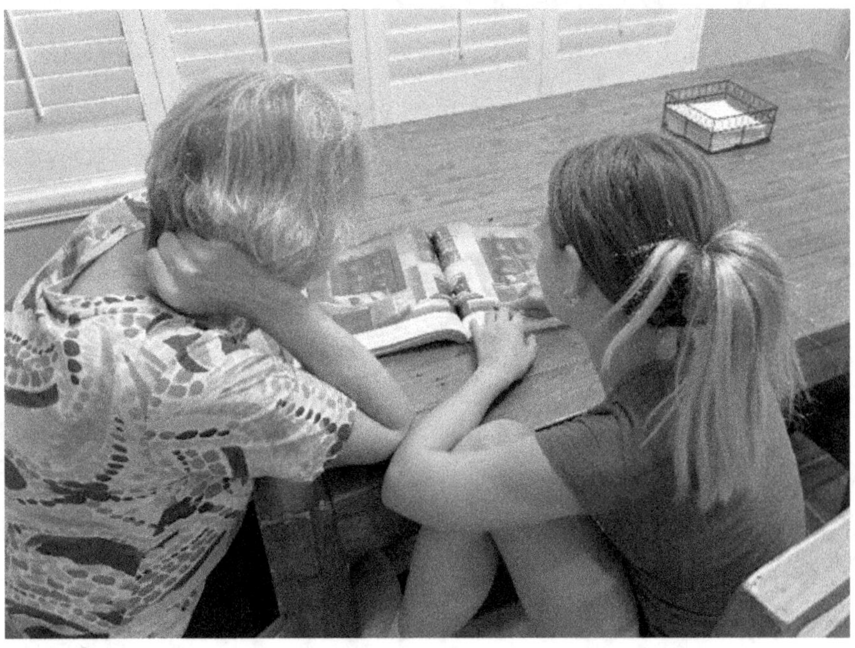

offering the kind of encouragement and understanding only a beloved grandparent can. We share a bond. As my Gram says, no matter what happens, we are linked in time for eternity. I want to share just a little bit of my life with you. I want you to be inspired by my story. Not because I think I am all that great or special, but because I want you to know if you are someone with ADHD or you love someone with ADHD, there is hope.

Gram and I hope you will discover the beauty in embracing your quirks and know that sometimes, it's ok to dance to a tune that no one else hears. Welcome to my world, where the story is just beginning...

My ADHD Life

In a world of constant motion,
Lives a girl with boundless emotion,

ADHD, her daily companion,
A unique rhythm, a different sensation.

Her thoughts like stars in a midnight sky,
Flicker and dance, never shy,

A kaleidoscope of ideas, so vast,
From the future to the distant past.

Her attention a fleeting butterfly,
Flitting from here to there, oh my,

But when she finds her passion's flame,
She soars, unstoppable, in her own name.

Impulsivity, a double-edged sword,
Sometimes leading to discord,

Yet in her spontaneity, you'll see,
A zest for life, wild and free.

She's not defined by her diagnosis,
But by her dreams and her doses

Of resilience, courage, and grace,
A girl with ADHD, embracing her space.

In a world that often seeks conformity,
She's a beacon of individuality,

With a heart that's strong and kind,
A girl with ADHD, one of a kind.

Chapter 1

Meet MG

Hi! I'm MG, and I'm in the 5th grade. My first and middle name is what I go by, not my initials. However, I will go by MG for this little book to maintain some privacy. My Gram says I have a signature name, which means it is unique.

Speaking of my Gram, she's my ghostwriter. In other words, we talk about Attention Deficit Hyperactivity Disorder (ADHD); she listens, observes, and writes. She also talks to my parents and observes how we interact around my attention deficit hyperactivity disorder. I need help organizing, forming letters, and putting my thoughts down on paper. My ghostwriter eliminates those problems. She's a great writer and organizer. My Gram has been with me my whole life and knows me well.

Some of this book will sound like me talking, and some will sound like my Gram. She says this is collaboration. Between the two of us, we hope to share with you my ADHD world.

There are also a lot of lists in this book. I do well with lists. This is a strategy I use to help me organize and make sense of my life. Plus, it's easier for the reader to remember. At least, it's easier for me to remember.

About Me

I want to tell you about my life and what it's like to have ADHD. Sometimes, people think I'm just a kid who can't focus, but there's a lot more to me than that. Sometimes I look dumb, but I am not. I am pretty smart, but there are holes in my brain. I have executive functioning problems. Something we will discuss a little later.

I'm a mystery. One of my teachers, who I like very much, told my mom that I look and act so "normally," so it's a shock to find out that I struggle academically. I am articulate, have a great sense of humor, and use irony and sarcasm well. I look like a normal kid…whatever that means. But looks can be deceiving and misleading, which is hard for me. I guess you would say, "I don't add up."

I have a sixth sense of the world. I can spot emotions in others from a mile away. My Gram says I am intuitive. I sound like a kid bound for med school. I'm not. I have a challenging mental health condition that plays tricks on me every day. I have to work hard to keep up and to have any success at all. Some days, I'm up to working that hard; others, I'm not. The result is that I wouldn't say I like school. I love my teachers and my friends; I hate the never-ending demands

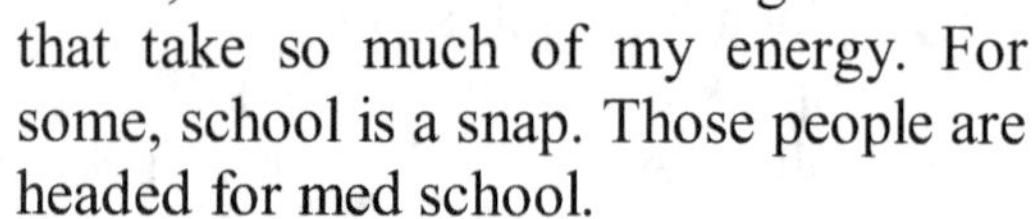

that take so much of my energy. For some, school is a snap. Those people are headed for med school.

I need some help with processing information. I can do it, but I need time and a lot of repetition. I also have trouble with fluency, so I don't always process information quickly. The processing and fluency problems go together to make my life difficult. For example, I can't recite the times tables from memory, yet, no matter how hard I try, or how threatening the state standards are. Threats don't work with my brain; in fact, threats only make things worse. What I need is time, patience and practice.

I don't cause problems or trouble like many kids with ADHD do. However, when I have to pay attention, I get bored, wiggle, and lose my focus. This happens when I'm not interested in something. I don't like math, so I have trouble paying attention. I love science, and I have no problem paying attention in science. See how that goes?

Focus

Children with Attention Deficit Hyperactivity Disorder (ADHD) often exhibit a unique pattern of attention and focus. It's indeed noticeable that they can concentrate intently on activities or subjects they are passionate about while struggling to maintain awareness on uninteresting or aversive tasks. This phenomenon can be attributed to several factors, both neurological and psychological. The following provides insight into the "I only pay attention to what I am interested in" phenomenon, and we will touch on some of this later.

Dopamine and Interest

One of the primary reasons why children with ADHD can focus on things they are interested in is related to dopamine, a neurotransmitter associated with motivation and reward. When they engage in activities they enjoy, their brains release more dopamine, making them feel good and more motivated to continue. This heightened dopamine release can enhance their ability to concentrate.

Hyper-focus

Children with ADHD can experience periods of hyper-focus on activities they are passionate about. During these episodes, they become completely absorbed in the task, often losing track of time. This intense focus can be so overpowering that they may neglect other responsibilities.

Intrinsic Motivation

Children interested in something are more likely to be intrinsically motivated. Intrinsic motivation is the desire to engage in an activity for its own sake rather than for external rewards or avoidance of punishment. This internal drive can help them maintain attention and effort.

Executive Functioning

ADHD is associated with challenges in executive functioning, which includes skills like organization, planning, and task initiation. When a task is uninteresting or perceived as tedious, children with ADHD may struggle to engage their executive functions effectively. In contrast, the novelty and appeal of something they're interested in can help them initiate and sustain their attention.

Emotional Regulation

Emotional regulation is often compromised in individuals with ADHD. Tasks they dislike or find frustrating can trigger negative emotions, further impairing their ability to focus. Conversely, activities they enjoy can evoke positive emotions, making concentrating easier.

Sensory Sensitivity

Some children with ADHD also have sensory sensitivities. Unpleasant sensory experiences, such as uncomfortable clothing or distracting noises, can make it exceedingly difficult for them to concentrate on tasks they dislike. In contrast, environments and activities aligned with their sensory preferences may facilitate better focus.

Task Relevance: Children with ADHD tend to be more focused when they perceive a task as immediately relevant or rewarding. If they understand how a particular activity relates to their interests or goals, they are likelier to engage with it. Conversely, tasks that seem pointless or disconnected from their interests may provoke resistance and inattention.

Understanding these dynamics is crucial for parents, educators, and caregivers. They underscore the importance of making tasks more engaging and relevant for children with ADHD. By tapping into their interests, providing structure, and helping them manage their emotions, it's possible to mitigate some of the challenges associated with focusing on less appealing tasks. Moreover, recognizing and celebrating their ability to hyper-focus on their passions can boost their self-esteem and overall well-being.

The person with ADHD is rewarded for what they like to do, so they can stick with it. However, they're not rewarded for what they don't want to do, so their focus fades.

I Love Sports!

Unfortunately, the subjects I hate are the subjects I could improve in. I do poorly in those subjects, which makes me hate them. It's like a merry-go-round.

I love sports and I'm good at them too. I'm a skinny, fearless ice hockey player. Hockey players aren't supposed to be thin, but I'm all muscle, and I can hit that puck with the speed of a pro…well, almost. I've played hockey for three years now; it's my life's love.

With hockey, I can be a star. I can get the answers right, make a goal, be a vital team member, and succeed. The more successful I am, the more successful I become. My Gram has talked to me about how other people with ADHD have used sports as a path to success. Many of us crave movement. Movement helps me think.

I can thank my mom for finding ice hockey for me and providing the opportunities and resources to succeed. Ice hockey is very expensive. The gear costs a lot of money, and I constantly need new equipment because I am growing. My mom and dad think ensuring I get what I need to play hockey is a priority.

I don't want to brag, but I think I'd do well at any sport. I was on a championship Cheer team for three years before I left for hockey. I was a base, which means I helped hold up the pyramid. Sports are my thing. School is not. Although I love my teachers, and they love me, I wouldn't say I like sitting and listening. Put a math concept on a hockey puck, and I could probably learn it! Well, maybe not.

I switched from Cheer to hockey for a couple of reasons. First, my mom took me to an ice hockey rink to introduce me to the ice. I loved it. Then, she signed me up for lessons and clinics. She put me in a recreation league when I did well and kept signing me up for more classes. I finally got good enough to be invited to play on an all-girls traveling team, but we moved before I could start.

Second, hockey is made up of a lot of friendly people. I haven't met one creep. The coaches are excellent, the kids are lovely, and the parents are amazing. There is nothing cutthroat. I know that runs counter to the free—for—all—you see on TV, but from my perspective, I have only experienced good people. No one gets mad, yells, or makes you feel stupid, even when you do something wrong.

Hockey players are usually gigantic, substantial people. Which means they don't usually do well with the gymnastics of conditioning. Seeing these beefy people trying to do the splits, handstands, or crab walks is hilarious. Their bulk gets in the way. So, these behemoths that I meet on the ice and who tower over me are left in knots when I can perform with the agility of a gymnast. They end up crying, "Uncle!"

By now, you might be wondering, "What exactly is ADHD?" Great question! ADHD stands for Attention Deficit Hyperactivity Disorder. It's like having a turbocharged brain with a short attention span. Think of it as having a brain constantly playing a game of musical chairs, except the chairs are your thoughts, and they're always on the move. My brain is like a never-ending rollercoaster and I'm just along for the ride. Sometimes, it's exhilarating; other times, it's frustrating and scary.

But here's the thing: ADHD isn't just about being the human embodiment of a fidget spinner. It's about uniquely seeing the world, like having a superpower. You know, like the ability to come up with a brilliant idea in the middle of math class or spot all the hidden treasures in a messy room that no one else can see.

So, welcome to my world, where the ordinary becomes extraordinary, and the chaos is just part of the daily routine!

Chapter 2

What is ADHD?

I want to explain what ADHD is and how it affects me. It's not just about being unfocused; it's about how my brain works differently. I'll introduce you to my brain, which sometimes feels like a rollercoaster. ADHD isn't just letters. It's like a puzzle; once you start putting the pieces together, you'll see it's more apparent than it seems.

Picture this: your brain is a busy city with thoughts rushing around like cars in traffic. In most people's brains, a traffic cop is telling those thoughts when to stop and go. But in my ADHD brain, that traffic cop sometimes takes a coffee break and forgets to return. So, what happens? Well, thoughts go zooming in all directions! Imagine trying to follow a hundred different TV shows at once. You'd get tangled up, right? That's like what happens in my head.

Types of ADHD

ADHD comes in different types. Yes! There's more than one! First, we have **hyperactive-impulsive subtype**. These kids have a turbocharged engine and can't sit still. You'll spot them doing cartwheels while waiting in line at the grocery store. They're human Tiggers from *Winnie the Pooh*, bouncing everywhere.

Then, there's **inattentive subtype**. These daydreamers can listen to a teacher drone on for hours and simultaneously think about their next scuba diving adventure.

Finally, there's a combined presentation subtype. The combined presentation is the most common subtype of ADHD. Individuals exhibit symptoms of both inattention and hyperactivity-impulsivity. They struggle with staying focused, being restless, and may act impulsively.

ADHD is a complex and heterogeneous condition, and individuals with the disorder may exhibit symptoms that vary in intensity and combination.

Let's dive deeper into the inattentive type of ADHD and how it impacts me. Remember, ADHD isn't one-size-fits-all. In my case, it's the inattentive type I have. Here is a general idea of what I deal with:

Mind the Daydreams
Imagine sitting in class while your teacher talks about fractions. It's like being in a spaceship heading for the moon, but instead of paying attention to the mission, your mind decides to explore distant galaxies of thoughts. That's me on an average school day. My mind loves to wander, and it often takes me on unexpected adventures when I should be focusing on math or science.

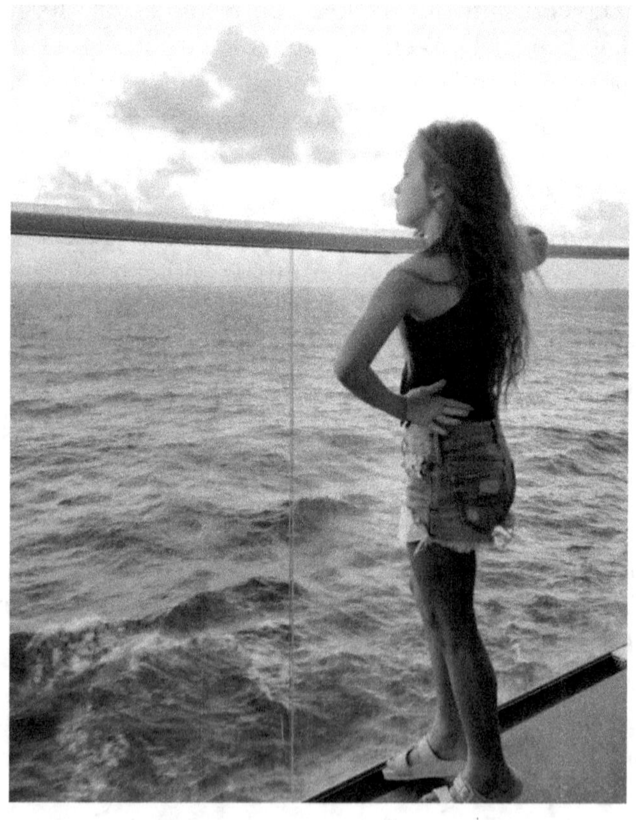

The Homework Black Hole

Ah, homework, the arch-nemesis of every student. It's like trying to tame a dragon with a rubber band. I can start with the best intentions, but before I know it, I've researched the history of rubber bands on the internet instead of solving math problems. Staying on track with homework can be a real challenge for an inattentive person like me.

Missing the Details

Ever heard the phrase, "The devil is in the details?" Sometimes, I feel like the devil is laughing at me, and I am unsure why. I need to catch essential details in instructions, which can be very difficult. I must hear, process, comprehend, and spit out an answer. This may take me much more time than my peers. My brain can skim over important information and get caught up in processing details, and all of a sudden everyone else in the class is putting their stuff away and heading for lunch. I might be able to finally get the answer but it takes me a long time.

The Waiting Game

Oh, patience, how hard for me! Waiting in line or sitting still can feel like trying to stop a tornado with your bare hands. It's not that I don't want to follow the rules; it's just that my body seems to have its own agenda.

Symptoms can strike at the most unexpected moments. But, you know what? It's not all bad news. There's a silver lining to this inattentive cloud. I might miss some details, but my brain's knack for seeing the big picture helps me develop creative solutions. My daydreams? Well, they've sparked some of my best inventions and imaginative adventures. And while I might misplace things, I'm also good at finding hidden treasures, like that shiny penny everyone else walked past.

It Can Be Hard to Relate

Understanding and empathizing with someone with ADHD, especially the inattentive type, can be challenging for those who don't have personal experience with the condition. Several factors contribute to this difficulty:

Invisible Nature
ADHD, especially the inattentive type, is often hidden. Unlike some physical disabilities or conditions with visible symptoms, ADHD doesn't manifest externally. This makes it harder for others to recognize the daily struggles individuals with ADHD face.

Stigma and Misconceptions
There are many misconceptions and stigmas surrounding ADHD. People may wrongly believe it is simply a lack of willpower or discipline. These misconceptions can lead to judgment and a lack of understanding.

Variable Symptoms
The symptoms of ADHD can vary widely from person to person. Some individuals may appear disorganized and forgetful, while others may excel in certain areas. This variability can lead to confusion and skepticism about the legitimacy of the condition.

Inconsistent Performance
People with ADHD may perform well in certain situations or on tasks they are passionate about, leading others to believe that they are not trying hard enough when they struggle with less exciting or more routine tasks.

Impaired Executive Functioning
ADHD often affects executive functions such as organization, time management, and planning. These difficulties can lead to missed deadlines and disorganization, or be misconstrued as laziness or irresponsibility.

Intangible Challenges

ADHD can cause internal challenges, such as difficulty focusing, racing thoughts, and emotional dysregulation. These experiences are not readily observable, making it challenging for others to grasp the extent of the challenges faced.

Frustration and Shame

Individuals with ADHD, predominantly inattentive, may feel frustrated and ashamed due to their struggles. They might work hard to hide their difficulties, making it even more challenging for others to understand their experiences.

Complex Diagnosis

ADHD is often diagnosed based on criteria and behavioral observations. This complexity can make it difficult for others to fully comprehend the diagnosis and its impact.

Improving Understanding

To improve understanding and support for individuals with ADHD inattentive type, it's essential to:

Educate

Provide information and resources about ADHD to family, friends, teachers, and colleagues to dispel myths and misconceptions.

Empathize

Try to put yourself in their shoes and recognize that their challenges are real, even if they aren't readily visible.

Listen and Communicate

Encourage open and honest communication with individuals with ADHD. Ask them about their experiences and needs.

Provide Structure and Support

Help with organization, time management, and strategies for managing ADHD symptoms.

Be Patient
Understand that setbacks may occur, and finding effective strategies and treatments may take time.

Advocate
Encourage individuals with ADHD to advocate for themselves and seek appropriate accommodations when necessary.

By fostering empathy, dispelling misconceptions, and offering support, we can create a more inclusive and understanding environment for individuals with ADHD, allowing them to thrive and reach their full potential. Having inattentive type ADHD isn't just about challenges; it's about finding the superpowers hidden within those challenges.

You may read my thoughts on my behavior more than once in this little book, but I want to stress that I am not a behavior problem. Poor behavior can be a massive issue for many kids with ADHD, regardless of the type. Being friendly and respectful and obeying the rules can work in my favor. The better I behave, the more friends I make, and the more teachers like me. I like being good because that means people will treat me well.

Home is a different story. Home is where my "demon" side can come out. Maybe all kids have a demon side, and it's just me being normal. My mom says I can get surly, make faces, and talk back. Still, I'm never, ever violent or aggressive. I know if I'm less than perfect, it's at home, never at school.

Sometimes, I'm unhappy with myself, and my lack of patience and many frustrations can consume me. I cry easily when I'm at home. Sometimes, it just gets to be too much. But that's only at home. Out in the world, I look just fine. Remember, this condition can be invisible.

ADHD is a disability. I'm protected under Section 504, part of a federal civil rights law, the Rehabilitation Act of 1973. I'll mention more of this later in my book. I have a 504 plan, which provides me with the accommodations I need to succeed in school.

Executive Functioning

ADHD can annihilate executive functioning skills. This is the motherboard of our brains. Executive functioning skills are higher-level cognitive processes that enable individuals to plan, organize, initiate, manage, and complete tasks. These skills are essential for everyday functioning and play a crucial role in achieving goals, solving problems, and adapting to new situations. Executive functioning skills are like the conductor of an orchestra, ensuring that all the individual instruments (cognitive processes) play in harmony to produce a well-organized and effective performance. Here are the critical components of executive functioning skills:

Inhibition

This skill allows individuals to control their impulses and resist distractions. It helps focus attention on relevant information and inhibiting irrelevant or impulsive responses. For example, it prevents people from blurting out an answer or resisting the temptation of checking their phone while working. The inhibition part of my brain works fine regarding my behavior out in the world. It's not as well functioning at home.

Working Memory

Working memory is the ability to hold and manipulate information in one's mind for short periods. It's crucial for following multi-step instructions, mental arithmetic, and decision-making. Think of it as your mental notepad where you jot down and manipulate information. Working memory is a massive problem for me. I have trouble holding information, especially numbers, in my brain, looking at them cognitively, and then doing what I am supposed to do with them.

Cognitive Flexibility

Cognitive flexibility enables individuals to adapt to changing situations, switch between tasks, and see things from different perspectives. It's essential for problem-solving and creativity.

This skill helps you "shift gears" mentally when, for example, switching from one subject to another or changing your approach to a problem. I have no mental or physical issues transitioning from topic to subject. I am good at looking at things differently, rejecting or accepting those ways, and moving on.

Planning and Organization

Planning involves setting goals, breaking them down into manageable steps, and creating a roadmap to achieve them. Organization means arranging and structuring tasks, time, and resources efficiently. These skills help you tackle complex projects, meet deadlines, and maintain order in your life. I am generally improving at organization, but I still need to complete homework without going in many different directions.

Initiation

Initiation is the ability to start tasks or activities independently. Many people with executive functioning challenges struggle with initiating studies, even if they know what needs to be done. It's like having the key to a car but not being able to turn it on and start driving. This is more of a problem at school with academics. I can create, build, imagine, and think about projects I want to work on at home. This is more of a hands-on or movement thing. For example, I love putting on shows with friends, and I am a master of recording those shows. I can plan, organize, and carry them out. I invent things and can work on a project from start to finish.

Emotional Regulation

Executive functioning skills include managing emotions and regulating situational reactions. This involves recognizing emotions, understanding their impact, and responding appropriately. Emotional regulation is essential for maintaining interpersonal relationships and making rational decisions. Out in the world, I am good at emotional regulation. At home, not so much.

Self-Monitoring

Self-monitoring involves evaluating, performing and adjusting strategies as needed. It helps individuals stay on track and make necessary corrections during tasks or activities. For instance, it allows you to assess your progress while studying and decide whether to change your approach. I can do this very well with hands-on projects and creative videos. I struggle with this at school.

Time Management

Time management estimates how long tasks will take, allocates time effectively, and prioritizes activities. It ensures you can meet deadlines and maximize your available time. This is a tricky one. My mom helps me with this a lot. I am ready for school on time; I have my stuff packed and ready to go. I hate being late. But I am only ten, and my mom has to keep my schedule of lessons and commitments.

Goal Setting

Setting clear and achievable goals is fundamental to executive functioning. This skill involves identifying your goals, determining the steps, and staying motivated to achieve those goals. I am all over this when it comes to hockey. I have big plans to visit different cities while on traveling teams; I want to see other parts of the United States. I love traveling, cruising, meeting new people, and seeing what the world offers. In school, I'm stuck. I still don't know what direction I'm headed.

Executive functioning skills mature gradually over time, with significant development occurring during childhood and adolescence. The older I get, the better I am at having it together. My current math teacher told my mom that I was organized. That's something my mom has never heard from a teacher before!

Effects of Poor Executive Functioning

Poor executive functioning skills can significantly impact the academic performance of a 5th-grade girl, affecting various aspects of her school life. Here's how:

Organization and Planning:
It's a process. I'm getting better.

Time Management
I do well after taking my medication in the morning. I CAN BE A MESS once I get home and my medication has worn off.

Task Initiation
Initiating tasks can be challenging. Even when I know what needs to be done, I can procrastinate or have difficulty starting assignments, particularly if they seem overwhelming or complex. I hate math and doing math homework at night is almost impossible.

Working Memory
Poor working memory can hinder the ability to follow multi-step instructions, comprehend complex concepts, and remember information from class to class. This can hinder understanding new topics and prevent me from reaching higher academic performance. My working memory is weak and has to work over time; this is exhausting and demoralizing and can cause me to give up on a learning task.

Task Completion
Difficulty in sustaining attention and staying on task may result in incomplete assignments or rushed work. I need help to stay with it during longer jobs. I can only do so much, and then my brain gives up.

Organization of Thoughts
I still need improvement with writing assignments. There's so much to think about and many moving parts to remember. My

Gram says I must use a keyboard and remember the writing mechanics.

Impulse Control

Impulsivity can lead to difficulties in classroom behavior, such as yelling out answers, interrupting others, or struggling to wait my turn. These behaviors can disrupt the learning environment and impact social relationships with peers and teachers. This is not me.

Emotional Regulation

Poor emotional regulation can affect my ability to handle frustration and stress effectively. This can result in me avoiding challenging tasks, which hurts my academic progress.

Test-Taking

During tests, executive functioning challenges cause me to have difficulties recalling information, organizing responses, and managing time effectively. This may lead to lower test scores and decreased confidence in my academic abilities. I'm a horrible test taker.

Homework Completion

Forget homework. When I get home from school, I'm done!

Note-taking

I need help to take notes. I fall apart between the mechanics of writing and figuring out what information is important enough to write down.

To me, school and its constant demands are overwhelming. I try. Sometimes I do well, but sometimes I need to do better. My abilities rest on how much gas is in my gas tank - energy. The gas helps me focus and sharpens my executive functioning skills. Medication, which I will talk about later, also helps me. But the drug wears off, my energy gets zapped after a full day of school, and my executive functioning skills suffer. I'm best in the morning after my medication and a good night's sleep. I can participate in hockey at night because it's very rewarding for me. However, trying to force myself to do math homework is almost impossible.

Why Is My Brain the Way It Is?

I want to touch on what happens in a person's brain with ADHD. ADHD, whether it's the inattentive type or combined type, is associated with specific patterns of brain activity and structure. While our understanding of the ADHD brain continues to evolve, here are some critical insights into the neurological aspects of inattentive ADHD.

Dopaminergic Dysfunction

One of the central characteristics of ADHD, including the inattentive type, is dysregulation in the brain's dopamine system. Dopamine is a neurotransmitter crucial in regulating attention, motivation, and reward. In individuals with ADHD, there may be lower-than-normal levels of dopamine or issues with dopamine receptor sensitivity, which can impact attention and impulse control.

Frontal Lobe Impairment

Brain imaging studies have shown that the frontal lobes, particularly the prefrontal cortex, tend to function differently in individuals with ADHD. The prefrontal cortex is responsible for executive functions, including decision-making, planning, organization, and working memory. In people with inattentive ADHD, this part of the brain may be less active or less developed, leading to difficulties in managing tasks and paying attention.

Structural Differences

Some research suggests that individuals with ADHD, including the inattentive type, may have structural brain differences. These differences can include a smaller brain volume, especially in attention and impulse control areas.

Cortical Arousal and Connectivity

Studies using functional MRI (fMRI) have shown that there can be differences in the activation patterns of various brain regions in people with ADHD. In the inattentive type, you may see reduced activity related to sustained attention and increased activity in areas associated with daydreaming or mind-wandering.

Default Mode Network (DMN)

The DMN is a network of brain regions active when the mind is at rest or engaged in internal thought processes, like daydreaming. In individuals with ADHD, including the inattentive type, the DMN may show activity when it should be suppressed during tasks requiring focused attention, contributing to distractibility.

Neurotransmitter Imbalance

Along with dopamine, other neurotransmitters like norepinephrine and serotonin also play roles in ADHD. Norepinephrine is involved in arousal and alertness, while serotonin influences mood and emotional regulation. Imbalances in these neurotransmitters can contribute to the symptoms of inattentive ADHD.

It's important to note that brain differences associated with ADHD do not indicate any moral failing or lack of intelligence. ADHD is a neurodevelopmental disorder, and these brain patterns are thought to be influenced by genetic and environmental factors. As mentioned in earlier, understanding these neurological aspects can help inform treatment strategies, often including behavioral therapy, medication, and lifestyle interventions, such as regular exercise and a structured routine. Additionally, the brain is highly adaptable, and interventions can help individuals with inattentive ADHD learn strategies to manage their symptoms effectively.

ADHD is a Neurodevelopmental Disorder

A neurodevelopmental disorder is a category of conditions characterized by developmental deficits or abnormalities in the structure or function of the nervous system, particularly the brain. These disorders typically manifest early in childhood and can impact an individual's cognitive, emotional, social, and behavioral functioning. Here are some key features and characteristics of neurodevelopmental disorders:

Onset in Early Development

Neurodevelopmental disorders are typically evident in early childhood, often before age three. Symptoms and developmental delays may become more apparent as a child grows and faces increasing cognitive and social demands.

Pervasive and Lifelong

These disorders tend to be pervasive, affecting multiple areas of a person's functioning. While symptoms may change and evolve, the underlying neurological differences persist into adulthood.

Neurobiological Basis

Neurodevelopmental disorders are rooted in neurobiological and genetic factors. Structural or functional abnormalities in the brain's development and functioning play a significant role in the manifestation of these conditions.

Heterogeneity

Neurodevelopmental disorders encompass various conditions with specific features and challenges. Along with ADHD, conditions like autism spectrum disorder (ASD), intellectual disabilities, and specific learning disorders (e.g., dyslexia) fall under this category. While they share some common characteristics, they also have unique traits and diagnostic criteria.

Functional Impairments
Individuals with neurodevelopmental disorders often experience significant functional impairments. Depending on the specific condition, these can include difficulties with communication, social interaction, motor skills, attention, learning, and emotional regulation.

Early Intervention
Early diagnosis and intervention are crucial for neurodevelopmental disorders. Early interventions, such as speech therapy, occupational therapy, behavioral therapy, and, in some cases, medication, can help mitigate the impact of these conditions and improve an individual's long-term outcomes.

Lifelong Management
While individuals with neurodevelopmental disorders may progress and acquire coping strategies, these conditions are usually lifelong. They often require ongoing support, accommodations, and therapies to help individuals reach their full potential and lead fulfilling lives.

Impact on Families
Neurodevelopmental disorders not only affect individuals, but also significantly impact their families and caregivers. Families may need to adapt their routines, seek specialized services, and provide extra support to help their loved ones thrive.

Social and Stigma Challenges
People with neurodevelopmental disorders may face social challenges and stigma due to their differences. Raising awareness, promoting acceptance, and educating about these conditions are essential to reducing stigma and fostering inclusivity.

Neurodevelopmental disorders are a group of conditions characterized by atypical brain development and functioning. They encompass a broad range of disorders with varying characteristics and challenges, but they all share the common feature of affecting an individual's development and functioning in multiple domains. Early diagnosis, intervention, and ongoing support are essential in helping individuals with neurodevelopmental disorders lead fulfilling lives.

Chapter 3

My Superpowers

Having ADHD isn't all bad. I'll share some cool things I can do because my brain works differently, like how I'm good at developing creative ideas and uniquely seeing the world.

I love, love, love science, and my dad does too. He's always up for science stuff. Recently, I captured a scorpion. He got me a fish bowl, and I investigated how to care for my new pet. He's very supportive of my off-the-wall projects.

One day he took my brother and me to dig up fossils and shark teeth. I loved it. I worked all day in the hot sun. My brother gave up after an hour and said, "This isn't for me."

I make all kinds of machines, and I love to invent things. My dad is always there to help me. He and I love to travel to thrift stores where we find incredible treasures. For example, Halloween is big for my dad. He covers the front lawn with every kind of Halloween icon imaginable. We even built a fog machine together out of thrift store parts!

ADHD Superpowers

The ADHD mind possesses a unique and often under-appreciated capacity for creativity and inventiveness. While attention deficit hyperactivity disorder is typically associated with focus and impulse control challenges, it also brings about a range of cognitive traits and thinking patterns that can fuel innovation and creativity. Some of the concepts in the list below appear elsewhere in the book, but, they are important enough to repeat. Here's how the ADHD mind can be creative and inventive:

Divergent Thinking

Individuals with ADHD excel in divergent thinking, which involves quickly generating many ideas and solutions. They often have a knack for seeing multiple perspectives on a problem, which can lead to innovative solutions. I need help with processing speed when dealing with information that could be more interesting to me. When I deal with topics I find fascinating, I'm quick.

Hyper-focus

While ADHD can lead to difficulties in sustaining attention, it can also result in episodes of hyper-focus. During these intense periods of concentration, individuals with ADHD become deeply absorbed in a task or topic of interest, often producing exceptional work or creative output.

High Energy and Enthusiasm

People with ADHD often have abundant energy and enthusiasm, which can be channeled into creative endeavors. Their enthusiasm can be infectious and inspire others to think creatively as well.

Risk-Taking

ADHD individuals may be more willing to take risks and explore unconventional approaches. This willingness to break the norm can lead to groundbreaking ideas and innovations.

Pattern Recognition

Some individuals with ADHD are talented at recognizing patterns and connections between seemingly unrelated ideas. This ability to make unexpected connections is a hallmark of creative thinking.

Out-of-the-Box Thinking

ADHD individuals are less constrained by traditional thought patterns and may be more open to exploring unconventional or out-of-the-box ideas.

Impulsivity

While impulsivity can be challenging, it can lead to spontaneous and creative ideas. An impulsive thought or action can sometimes spark innovative solutions or artistic expressions.

Multitasking Abilities

Contrary to the belief that individuals with ADHD cannot multitask, some are adept at juggling multiple tasks simultaneously. This ability can be harnessed to approach problems from various angles and generate creative solutions.

Passion and Intensity

Individuals with ADHD often have intense interests and passions. This intense focus on a particular topic or project can lead to profound exploration and creative breakthroughs.

Adaptability

The ADHD mind is often highly adaptable and can quickly switch between tasks or ideas. This adaptability can be an asset when working on complex, multifaceted creative projects.

My dad is very talented in fixing things and figuring out mechanical things. My Gram encourages him to teach me because number 1. I love that kind of thing, and number 2. My Gram is trying to find a career path for me. My dad thinks this may be premature, but my Gram is relentless. She's a long-range planner. She's also realistic. She knows I probably won't be the valedictorian of my graduating high school class or write the Great American novel. She also knows I'm intelligent and is determined to match my abilities with life skills that will support me.

My Gram is a career woman. She wants me to be financially independent and be able to take care of myself when I grow up. She also wants me to be happy. She's like a heat-seeking missile when it comes to searching for that perfect mix of what I can be good at and what will make me happy. Sometimes, she is a little intense.

I'm curious about all kinds of things. My dad will take off on that, and we'll work together on projects. Sometimes I like it, and sometimes I don't. Mostly, however, I like being with my dad. We watch science shows on TV and, sometimes, we'll try the presented projects. We love making slime, but my mom has announced that there will be no more slime in the house.

My Gram says my dad is good at being spontaneous. He will, all of a sudden, decide that we need to go out and watch the sunset. I love it. He knows about stars and galaxies, and we talk about what is happening in space.

I love playing board games; I can be very competitive…especially with my brother. I learn best when I'm moving. I know learn with hands-on projects. If school subjects were board games, I'd do better.

ADHD has its fair share of strengths and unique qualities that can be advantageous. Here are some of the more positive aspects of having ADHD and examples of how they pertain to me.

Hyper-focus
While I may struggle with attention in some areas when something genuinely captures my interest, I can dive into it with incredible intensity. This hyper-focus allows me to become an expert in my passions and accomplish tasks others might find difficult.

Creativity
I have a remarkable ability to think outside the box. I see connections and possibilities that others might overlook. I can be an excellent problem solver and innovator.

Resilience
Managing ADHD can be challenging, but fosters resilience. I've learned to adapt to my unique way of processing the world, which can translate into valuable life skills such as adaptability, perseverance, and the ability to handle change effectively.

High Energy
I have boundless energy, which can be a tremendous asset in various situations. I have a lot of enthusiasm and vivacity

regarding group projects, sports, and social activities. This makes me motivated and excited.

Empathy
I'm highly empathetic. In social situations, I can think quickly and react to changing events. I'm an excellent listener and offer friends emotional support when needed.

Fast Thinkers
I have an agile mind, which means I can process information in ways that provide me with alternatives to problems. In my case, I'm a slow processor, but that doesn't mean I can't come up with great ideas. I need time.

Adaptability:
I have a flexible thinking style when comfortable, which lets me quickly adapt to new environments and situations. I'm open to trying new things and embracing change, which can lead to exciting opportunities.

Spontaneity
Life with ADHD can be an adventure with unexpected twists and turns. I can be spontaneous and see them as opportunities for excitement and growth.

Natural Leaders
I have high energy and enthusiasm and can be a leader among my friends. When I'm comfortable, I can think clearly and make good decisions.

Positive Outlook
I try to have an optimistic outlook on life. I focus on what's possible rather than dwelling on limitations, which can be infectious and motivating to those around me.

Introducing Chuckles

ADHD is like having a unique set of tools in your utility belt. It's all about learning to harness these strengths and manage the challenges. There are significant limitations to having ADHD, but there are also opportunities.

One of my superpowers is art—the drawing and painting kind. My mom put me in art classes last year, and I loved it. It opened a whole new world and made me feel calm and helped me express myself.

I love dogs, and until recently, we had an English bulldog named Chuckles. My mom called him Charles, and my Gram called him Chuck. He answered to anything. He was a very versatile dog and very smart. He was quite sweet and always in the mix of the family. He loved my dad, and my dad loved him. He would sit by my dad's side and, if my dad was unhappy about anything, would lick him. I think that was his way of comforting my dad.

Next to my dad, Chuckles loved my Gram. He would sit as close to her as possible and lean on her…all 70 pounds of him. If you've ever seen an English bulldog, you know that they're low to the ground, have a terrible under bite, and weigh as much as a boat anchor. Chuckles was a good eater; that's my Gram's way of saying he ate everything in his path and then some. He loved everyone in our family, but could be pushy around other dogs. He was never pushy around us.

Chuckles also passed a lot of gas. He walked around in a constant cloud of stink that could empty a room in 5 seconds. He didn't ever seem to mind his far-reaching flatulence. I think he thought it was one of his most endearing qualities.

One day, my dad noticed a small mass on Chuckles' side. He took him to the vet. The vet said it was cancer. The vet told my dad that Chuckles could stay with us as long as he was comfortable and not in pain.

We were all very sad, but we pushed our sadness out. We ignored the fact that Chuckles was dying. My dad didn't accept it. He was prepared to do whatever it took to heal Chuckles. Ultimately, he decided that putting Chuckles through any rigorous treatment would be awful for him.

We waited and pretended that Chuckles was okay and made sure he wasn't in any pain. One day, we came home, and Chuckles had died. My brother lay down beside him. Our whole family went into mourning; especially my dad. When Chuckles left, he took a big piece of our hearts. We all handled Chuck's death differently.

My dad was very quiet, my brother and I cried and cried. My mom tried to be supportive of all of us, but she felt pretty bad too. My dad got a shovel and dug a big hole in our backyard. He placed Chuckles in the hole. We all stood and watched silently. The next days and weeks were tough. Chuckles was an important member of our family. I made this picture of Chuckles for my dad for Christmas.

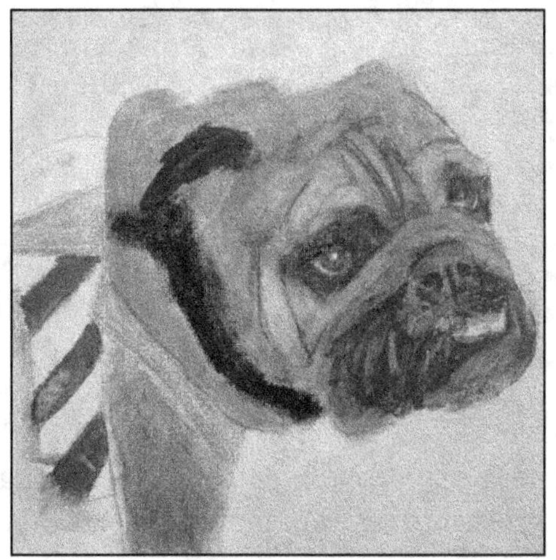

"Chuckles" by MG

Art Can Be a Superpower

Art can be a powerful tool to help people with inattentive type ADHD. While it might not directly address all the challenges associated with ADHD, it can provide significant benefits that complement other coping strategies and interventions. Art can be constructive for individuals with inattentive type ADHD. It would be best if you had focus and concentration to complete art projects. You have to pay attention to detail. I've worked on pictures for hours, deciding on perspective, color, and arrangement. This has helped my concentration. Although, it's easy to concentrate when doing something I love.

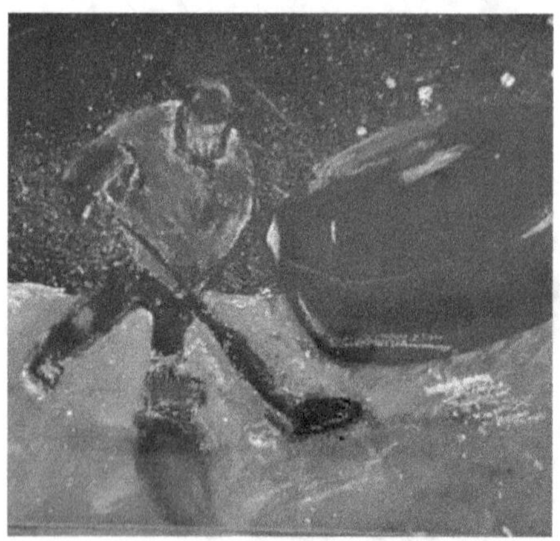

"Ice Hockey" by MG

Art can also reduce stress and be very therapeutic. I get lost in my art projects and feel very calm. It's like meditating, and it reduces anxiety. I can't feel overwhelmed when I'm working on an art project. It's my Zen time.

Art can also improve executive functioning skills: Art projects often involve planning, organization, and sequential thinking. Whether it's deciding on colors, materials, or the order of steps, these activities naturally stimulate and strengthen executive functioning skills, which can be challenging for individuals with inattentive type ADHD. Completing an art project provides a sense of accomplishment and pride. When I finish an art project, I get a lot of praise and appreciation. I feel pride and satisfaction.

Art can be an alternative means of communication. I can draw my emotions and share my thoughts via my art. Art allows me to enhance my creativity and problem-solving skills. The creative process encourages me to think outside the box, explore new possibilities, and develop innovative solutions. These skills can be transferable to other areas where creative problem-solving is required. Art also gives me a sense of control. It allows me to choose my materials, colors, and subject matter, giving me a sense of ownership over my work.

Art can be a constructive way to combat boredom. I can be quickly bored, but when I start working on an art project, my mind calms and focuses, and I enjoy myself. It also helps me improve my patience because you can't hurry through an art project. Art can be a social activity because I take art classes and attend workshops and art camps.

Art builds resilience. Art encourages experimentation and learning from mistakes. Art can teach resilience by showing that making mistakes and trying again is okay. Art helps with regulating emotions. It provides a structured, non-judgmental space to channel my energy positively.

Art can be a therapeutic and empowering outlet for individuals with inattentive type ADHD. It offers a range of cognitive, emotional, and social benefits that complement other strategies for managing ADHD symptoms. Whether painting, drawing, sculpting, or any other creative endeavor, art can be valuable in helping individuals harness their unique strengths and talents.

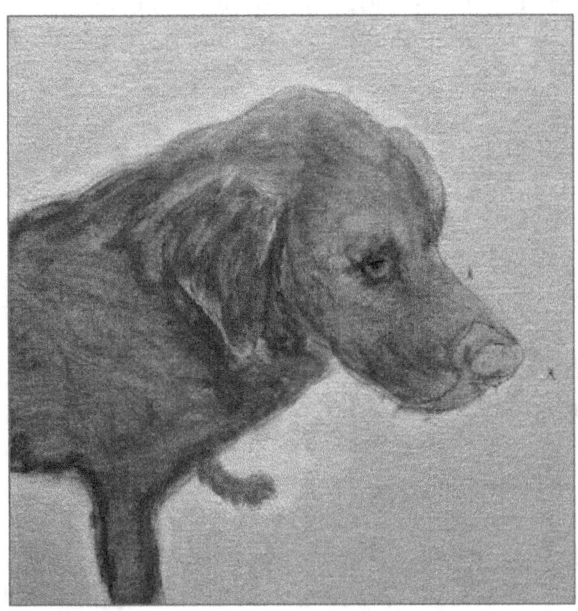

"Chester" by MG

Chapter 4

Challenges at School

School can be tricky sometimes. Let me tell you about my struggles with paying attention in class, finding motivation, and doing homework.

Twice-Exceptional

First and foremost, kids with ADHD are not dumb. Many of us have a high IQ, and some have a very high IQ. Kids that have high IQs and ADHD can be "twice exceptional." People do not understand how you can be smart and do poorly in school. Unfortunately, it's easy.

Being twice-exceptional refers to individuals with exceptional intellectual or creative abilities and one or more disabilities or challenges. When someone with ADHD is also identified as gifted or exceptionally intelligent, it presents a unique set of circumstances and opportunities. Here's a closer look at what it means to be twice-exceptional with ADHD inattentive type and how it can impact a person's life:

Intellectual Gifts

Twice-exceptional individuals often demonstrate high intelligence, creativity, or talent levels in one or more areas. They may excel in mathematics, science, the arts, or problem-solving.

Unique Strengths

Gifted individuals with ADHD inattentive type may possess unique strengths, including creativity, out of the box thinking, and the ability to make unexpected connections between ideas.

Challenges with Executive Functioning

Executive functioning skills, such as organization, time management, and planning, are often difficult for individuals with ADHD. These challenges can affect their ability to translate their intellectual potential into academic or professional success.

Uneven Performance

Twice-exceptional individuals may exhibit uneven academic performance. They can excel in areas of interest and struggle in tasks that require sustained attention or organization.

Frustration and Self-Esteem

Balancing giftedness with ADHD can lead to feelings of frustration and lowered self-esteem. Individuals may wonder why they excel in some areas but struggle with seemingly basic tasks.

Misdiagnosis or Under-identification

ADHD symptoms may be masked or overlooked in gifted students because they compensate for their challenges with intelligence. This can lead to under-identification or misdiagnosis, delaying the provision of necessary support.

Individualized Support

Recognizing and understanding the unique combination of giftedness and ADHD is essential for providing adequate support. Individualized educational plans, accommodations, and interventions can help these individuals thrive.

Embracing Differences

Embracing one's differences and advocating for tailored support is essential. It's important to understand that being twice-exceptional is not a contradiction, but a unique blend of strengths and challenges.

Resilience and Creativity

Many twice-exceptional individuals develop resilience and creative problem-solving skills as they navigate the complexities of their condition. They often find innovative ways to overcome challenges.

Supportive Environment

A supportive environment at home and school is crucial. Parents, teachers, and mentors can play a significant role in helping these individuals understand their strengths and develop strategies to manage their challenges.

Encouraging Passions

Encouraging twice-exceptional individuals to pursue their passions and interests can provide a sense of purpose and motivation to overcome obstacles.

Being twice-exceptional with ADHD and giftedness is a unique journey. It requires a nuanced approach to education, support, and self-understanding. With the right resources, encouragement, and a focus on strengths, these individuals can harness their exceptional abilities and navigate the challenges of ADHD to achieve their full potential.

Having a high IQ and having ADHD are not mutually exclusive. IQ measures cognitive abilities, such as problem-solving, logical reasoning, and abstract thinking, while ADHD primarily affects attention, focus, and impulse control. Here's how it's possible to have both a high IQ and ADHD:

Diverse Cognitive Abilities

IQ tests assess a wide range of cognitive abilities. While ADHD may impact attention and executive functions, it doesn't necessarily affect all aspects of cognitive functioning. Many people with ADHD excel in certain areas of intelligence, such as creativity, pattern recognition, or out of the box thinking.

Compensatory Strategies

Individuals with ADHD often develop compensatory strategies to cope with their challenges. They may use their intellectual strengths to find innovative solutions to problems, enabling them to overcome the difficulties associated with ADHD.

Hyper-focus

ADHD individuals can experience hyper-focus, a state where they become deeply engrossed in a task of interest. During these episodes, their heightened concentration and intense focus can lead to exceptional performance, especially in areas they're passionate about.

Diverse Interests

ADHD individuals tend to have various interests and passions. This diversity of interests can lead them to explore different fields, accumulate knowledge, and excel in multiple areas, contributing to a high IQ.

Treatment and Support

Many individuals with ADHD receive treatment and support, which can help them better manage their symptoms. With appropriate interventions, they can harness their intelligence more effectively and ease the challenges associated with ADHD.

It's essential to recognize that intelligence is multifaceted and cannot be solely determined by an IQ test. ADHD, like any other condition, affects individuals differently, and many factors, including genetics, environment, and personal motivation, play a role in cognitive development. The presence of ADHD should not be viewed as a limitation, but as a unique aspect of an individual's neurodiversity. With the proper support and strategies, individuals with ADHD can leverage their intelligence to achieve their goals and excel in various parts of life.

My School Challenges

Individuals face many school challenges with inattentive type ADHD.

Focusing in Class

One of the most apparent challenges for inattentive type ADHD students is maintaining focus during class lectures. My mind may drift while the teacher explains a lesson, making absorbing the information difficult. This can lead to missed details and lower comprehension of the subject matter. As I mentioned, I wouldn't say I like math, so listening to anything math-related is especially difficult. I just don't care.

Staying on Task

Inattentive type ADHD students often struggle to stay on task. Again, this is especially true when we have no interest in the subject. Even with the best intentions, I may become easily distracted by external stimuli, classmates, or my thoughts, making it challenging to complete assignments efficiently.

Time Management

Time management can be a significant hurdle. We must pay more attention to how long tasks take to complete, leading to rushed work or missed deadlines. In my case, I can also get lost in hyper-focus and losing track of time. I have little left to give when I get home, so I put off doing homework, and then the night slips away.

Listening Skills

Effective listening in class is essential for learning. We might need support with instructions so we don't miss important details or need help following verbal explanations. I have much better listening skills if I'm in a class I like or at hockey practice.

Forgetfulness

My working memory can be a challenge. I must remember to turn in assignments and bring necessary materials to class. Sometimes I even forget why I entered a room! This forgetfulness can lead to frustration and lower academic performance.

Test Anxiety
I can't ever take computerized tests successfully. I've gotten so I don't care.

Homework Struggles
Completing homework assignments can be a prolonged process. I might start and stop multiple times, leading to extended study hours. Additionally, maintaining focus on homework can be challenging, making it feel like an uphill battle.

Written Assignments
Writing assignments can be particularly demanding. I need help with just writing. The mechanics of writing could be better for me. I also need help with coherently organizing my thoughts.

While these school challenges are natural, it's important to remember that inattentive type ADHD students also possess a range of strengths and talents.

How IQ and ADHD Coexist
I want to return to something I said about my processing and fluency problems. I had a psychological evaluation last spring. My mom and dad wanted to know my strengths and weaknesses. My parents have always told me I am intelligent, but I've had so many academic struggles I didn't believe them.

I was tested in two separate sessions by a psychologist. She was very nice. I don't want to get into all the numbers she got on me, but I want to say that my General Ability Index (GAI) was 118. This places me at the 88th percentile based on her assessment. That means I am more intelligent than 88 percent of the people my age. In addition, the psychologist noted that this was a low estimate of my cognitive abilities. She felt my ADHD was interfering with my performance.

Having a higher IQ and struggling in school with ADHD is not uncommon. It's important to understand that IQ measures cognitive abilities and potential, while ADHD primarily affects a person's executive functions, such as attention, impulse control, and organization.

IQ measures a person's cognitive abilities, including problem-solving, reasoning, memory, and overall intellectual potential. Children with a high IQ typically have solid intellectual capabilities and may excel in tasks requiring abstract thinking, creativity, and critical reasoning.

Despite their high cognitive abilities, children with ADHD may face several challenges in an academic setting, such as, difficulty with organization, inconsistent performance, procrastination (difficulty initiating and completing tasks,) and impaired executive functions. External factors such as the school environment, teachers and teaching methods as well as, treatment and support play important roles, as well.

A high IQ and ADHD can coexist because IQ measures cognitive potential, while ADHD affects attention, impulsivity, and organization. Children with ADHD may struggle in school despite their high IQ due to challenges related to executive functions. The key is in finding tailored support and interventions to address their specific needs in the academic setting.

Hyper-focus

I've mentioned hyper-focus more than once in this book and want to elaborate on it more here. Hyper-focus is a fascinating aspect of ADHD, including the inattentive type, characterized by an intense and unwavering concentration on a specific task or activity. It contrasts the common perception that individuals with ADHD have difficulty maintaining attention. Here's an in-depth look at hyper-focus and how it manifests in kids with ADHD inattentive type.

Intense Concentration
Hyper-focus involves an extreme form of concentration. When kids with ADHD inattentive type experience hyper-focus, they become completely absorbed in a particular activity, often to the exclusion of everything else. They may lose track of time and be oblivious to their surroundings.

Selective Focus
Hyper-focus occurs on activities or tasks that captivate a child's interest or passion. It's as if they can select what they hyper-focus on, typically gravitating toward subjects or projects that align with their intrinsic motivations.

Sustained Attention
During a hyper-focus episode, a child with ADHD inattentive type can maintain their focus for an extended period, often longer than their typical attention span for less engaging tasks. This ability to sustain attention can lead to impressive productivity and depth of understanding in the chosen area of interest.

Immersion
Hyper-focus is like diving into a deep pool of interest. Kids can immerse themselves so completely in the activity that it becomes a primary mental and emotional focus. This immersion often results in high-quality work and creative output.

Lack of Awareness
While in a state of hyper-focus, children with ADHD inattentive type may be unaware of their surroundings, neglecting responsibilities, or even ignoring basic needs like eating or sleeping. This can sometimes lead to frustration from parents or teachers who struggle to redirect their attention.

Difficulty Shifting Focus

Once a hyper-focus episode begins, it can be challenging for the child to switch their attention to other tasks or responsibilities. They may resist interruptions and become frustrated when disengaging from their chosen activity.

Productive Outcomes

Hyper-focus can result in impressive accomplishments. Children may complete complex projects, create art, or excel academically when they're in a state of hyper-focus.

Emotional Attachment

Kids often form a strong emotional attachment to the activity or subject of their hyper-focus. This emotional connection can further fuel their dedication and motivation.

Variable Occurrence

Hyper-focus episodes are not constant and can be unpredictable. A child may struggle to focus on mundane tasks but display hyper-focus when engaged in something they find genuinely captivating.

Utilizing Hyper-focus

Parents and educators can leverage a child's hyper-focus by helping them explore their interests and incorporating them into learning or task completion. It's an opportunity to enhance their strengths and use their focused periods to their advantage.

While hyper-focus can be a remarkable asset, striking a balance is essential. Children with ADHD should also receive support in developing strategies to manage their attention and tasks that require less intrinsic motivation. Harnessing the power of hyper-focus while addressing the challenges associated with ADHD can help these children thrive academically and creatively.

I will dedicate another book to discussing my academic problems, their meaning, and how they impact me. But, for now, understand that I am not dumb…not dumb at all.

Chapter 5

Friendship Adventures

Friends are important to me, and I do very well socially. I've made and kept friends from different places I've been to. I've been to 2 schools and still have many friends from the first school. We call, text, and chat.

This past spring, my family went on a cruise to Alaska, and I made many friends at the Kid's Club on board. We're still communicating in a group chat. They're from all over the United States.

Some kids with ADHD have problems making friends. I don't. I have some fantastic friends that I hope to keep forever. They are lovely people. If my inattentiveness is on one end of the spectrum of being me, my social appropriateness is on the other end. I think I "hit it out of the ballpark" in the friend department. One reason is that I know how to read people. Like my Gram says, "Read your audience."

Reading people, often called "social intelligence" or "emotional intelligence," is a valuable skill that involves understanding and interpreting non-verbal cues, verbal communication, and behavioral patterns to gain insights into a person's thoughts, emotions, and intentions. Here are some tips on how to read people effectively.

Observe Non-Verbal Cues

Body Language
Attention to body posture, gestures, and facial expressions. Crossed arms indicate defensiveness, while an open stance may suggest receptivity.

Eye Contact
The eyes can reveal a lot about a person's emotions and level of engagement. Prolonged eye contact often indicates interest or sincerity.

Facial Expressions

Recognize basic facial expressions like happiness, sadness, anger, and surprise. Micro-expressions, fleeting words that occur in less than a second, can provide deeper insights.

Tone of Voice

Listen to their speech's tone, pitch, and speed. Changes in fashion can indicate shifts in emotion or emphasis on specific points.

Pay Attention to Verbal Communication

Content

Analyze what a person is saying. Are they providing detailed information or being vague? Are they using positive or negative language?

Consistency

Note if their verbal and non-verbal cues align. Inconsistencies might indicate hidden emotions or deceit.

Active Listening

Show that you're engaged and interested in their words. This encourages open communication and may reveal more about their thoughts and feelings.

Consider Context

Environmental Factors

Take into account the setting and circumstances. Someone may act differently in a professional meeting compared to a social gathering.

Cultural Differences
Cultural norms can influence communication styles and body language. What's considered polite or rude can vary significantly between cultures.

Ask Open-Ended Question
Encourage people to share more by asking questions that require thoughtful responses rather than simple "yes" or "no" answers. This can help you gain deeper insights into their perspectives.

Empathize and Connect
Put yourself in their shoes and try to understand their point of view. This can help you connect on a more emotional level and build rapport. Show empathy by acknowledging their feelings and validating their experiences.

Notice Behavioral Patterns
Observe recurring behaviors and reactions in different situations. People often exhibit consistent patterns in their responses to various stimuli.

Be Mindful of Your Own Biases
Recognize that your beliefs, values, and biases can influence your interpretations. Try to approach interactions with an open mind.

Trust Your Intuition
Sometimes, your gut feeling can provide valuable insights. If something feels off or inconsistent, it might be worth exploring further.

Practice Patience
Developing the ability to read people takes time and practice. Be patient with yourself and others as you refine this skill.

Seek Feedback
Ask for feedback from trusted friends or mentors on your ability to read people. They may provide valuable insights and guidance for improvement.

Reading people is not about making assumptions or judgments but fostering better communication, understanding, and empathy. As you become more adept at reading people, you'll enhance your interpersonal relationships and ability to effectively navigate social and professional situations.

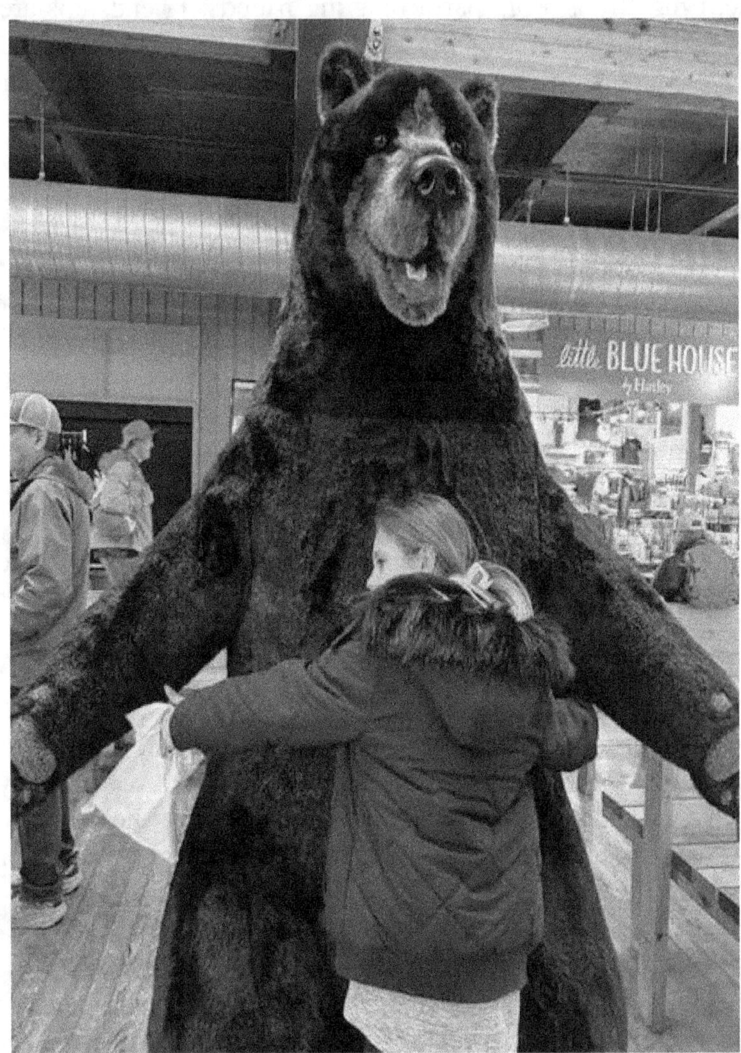

Many kids, not just those with ADHD, miss the boat. I'm friendly and kind. I don't make fun of people, but have a great sense of humor without being mean or nasty. If someone's being disagreeable, I avoid them. At the same time, I have no problem standing up for myself when necessary. So far, it's all worked for me socially.

I also have a lot of empathy for people. That's part of reading people, understanding their feelings, and appreciating them. I like people. Empathy is a big part of having friends. Friendships are like the secret sauce that makes life extra delicious; for kids with ADHD, they're even more critical. Having good friends isn't just about fun and games; it's crucial to thriving with ADHD. Let's dive into why friendships are so vital for kids like us.

Understanding and Acceptance
True friends see you for who you are, quirks and all. They understand that sometimes you might need to be more mindful or focused, but they accept you just as you are. Having friends who get you can be incredibly comforting and reassuring.

Emotional Support
Life can be a rollercoaster, and sometimes ADHD can make it feel even crazier. Friends are like seatbelts on that rollercoaster. They're there to hold you steady during the ups and downs. You can lean on them when discussing your challenges or sharing your victories.

Social Skills Practice
Friendships provide the perfect playground for practicing social skills. Whether taking turns, listening actively, or resolving conflicts, interacting with friends helps you fine-tune these skills. It's like your personal social skills training camp!

Building Self-Esteem
Good friends boost your self-esteem. They remind you of your strengths, celebrate your achievements, and offer encouragement when feeling down. With friends, you'll feel like you can conquer the world.

Collaborative Learning

Friendships offer unique learning opportunities. When you work on group projects or explore shared interests with friends, you learn from each other. They might introduce you to new hobbies or ways of thinking you have yet to consider.

Fun and Laughter

Laughter is like a superpower in its own right. Friends bring joy, fun, and a dose of silliness into your life. They're your adventure partners, creating unforgettable memories that blast life.

Reducing Loneliness

ADHD can sometimes make you feel like you're on an island, but friends are like bridges connecting you to the mainland. They ward off loneliness and give you a sense of belonging. Even on your most challenging days, knowing you have friends who care about you can make a difference.

Shared Experiences

Having friends means you're not alone in your ADHD journey. You can swap stories, share strategies, and offer each other valuable insights. It's like having a support group right there with you.

Positive Influence

Good friends can be positive role models. They inspire you to work on your weaknesses and celebrate your strengths. You'll find yourself adopting their good habits and values, which can help you manage your ADHD more effectively.

Unconditional Love

Lastly, friends offer something precious: unconditional love. They love you for who you are, regardless of your ADHD challenges. That kind of love is like a superpower, providing strength and comfort in even the most challenging times.

I get accommodations and extra help in school. My friends see that. Most of my friends have no problems in school; they excel. No one has ever made fun of me or made me feel stupid. They have never questioned me or acted superior around me. That's important. No kid wants to feel like the class dummy. My friends treat me like I'm smart. That's a massive piece of friendship: never looking down on your friends and always respecting them.

Chapter 6

Family Support

My family plays a significant role in helping me manage my ADHD and getting through life. I'll introduce you to my parents and how they support me. Plus, you'll meet my brother, who sometimes drives me crazy.

My dad was brought up on the theory that it is okay to spank kids; I think he got spanked a lot. He doesn't abide by the spanking theory with me or my brother. He used to, but he found out it didn't do much good and caused more problems than cured.

It goes back to reading your audience. My dad is thoughtful and kind and not a bully. He knows that if he tries to control us physically, it won't teach us anything but to fear him. Fear and love have a hard time living together, especially between a parent and a child. At some point, you have to talk it out and listen. I make many mistakes, but I wouldn't go to my dad for help if I thought he would hurt me verbally or physically. Don't get me wrong, he disapproves of my behavior when necessary, but knows I won't trust him if he is unfair. Kids have a real sense of fairness and justice. If that's compromised, relationships start to break down.

My dad's a lot like me. He seems to understand that when I'm bad at home, I'm suffering inside. It's hard to explain, but it goes back to this: if I'm going to have behavior problems, it can only be at home, never out in the world.

My mom is my rock. I'm most difficult with her. She bends backward to make me happy, and I often lack gratitude and appreciation. She's always surprising me with cool things. We're not rich, but she and my dad make sure my brother and I have what we need and then some.

My mother is beautiful. That's what my dad calls her all the time, "beautiful." People say I'm beautiful. I don't think my mom and I look alike, but it makes me happy when people say we do.

My mom and my Gram guide the ship that is called my life. Once my Gram has investigated something, she will talk with my mom, dad, and Papa. My mom takes the lead and, after talking with my dad, if she agrees with Gram, will be the one to make the appointments and schedules. That doesn't mean that my dad isn't involved. He is…very. But he works many hours, and my mom works part-time. Combining my mom and dad's brains with my Gram and Papa is pretty unbeatable.

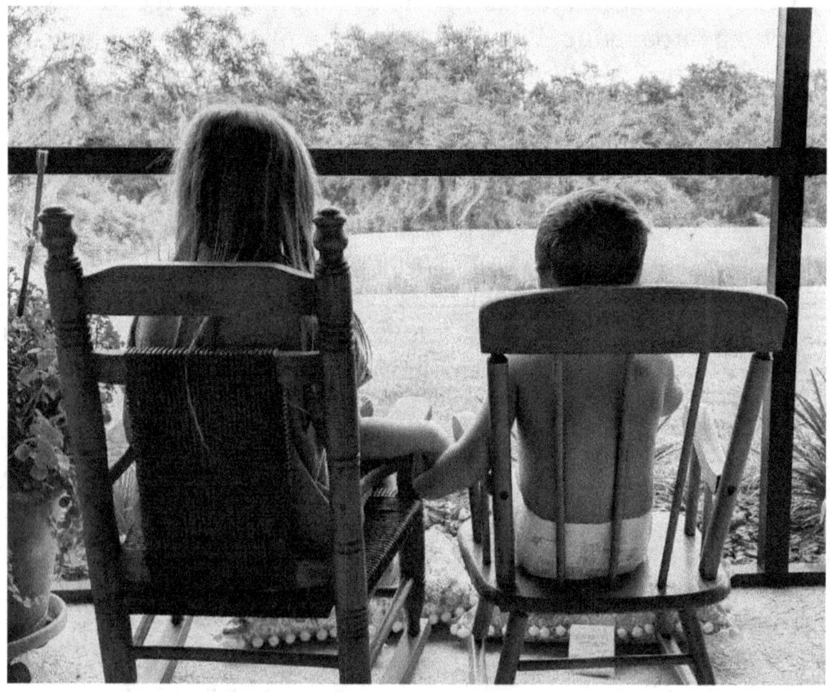

My brother's two years younger than me. He's nicer to me than I am to him. He drives me crazy. He's a lot more careful than I am and a lot more sensitive. My mom thinks he will work for OSHA when he gets big. He is very, very careful and obeys all the rules. You don't have to tell him twice. He hates any sports where he might get hurt. My parents put him in flag football last spring, and he said the experience traumatized him. My parents were always at his practices and games and said everyone was very friendly to him.

My Papa is my mother's father. He's essential to me. I think I'm his favorite, although he says he doesn't have a favorite. He's probably the only person who can work with me in math and make me understand it. He's patient, calm, supportive, and never gives up on me. I call him when I need new hockey gear. He always says yes. He's my silent advocate. He is always on my side. He's talking about taking flying lessons. If he does, he said I can take them, too.

My Gram is my mother's mom and constantly pushes me to "strive" for all good things. She puts me in lessons. I love art lessons, but I don't like swimming lessons. She told me I could quit swimming when I could swim perfectly the length of the pool twice. I was very irritated with her. I can swim, but she doesn't think I can swim well enough. She thinks my swimming looks like a splashing mess.

Gram is apprehensive about my academic future. What kind of school would be best? I will talk about this at another time. Since I'm in the last year of elementary, everyone is thinking about what the best school would be for me for next year. Virtual? Charter? Public? Homeschool? My Gram will investigate, research, interview, and talk everyone else in my family to death about this decision.

My Gram will spend her last dime on my brother and me if she thinks it will help us. My Papa and Gram are retired and have built their dream home. However, they sold that dream home and will move close to us. We are at the top of the list of what is important to them.

My Gram and my dad are very different, but very much the same. My Gram couldn't hammer a nail in a piece of wood. My dad could build a house from scratch. But they love to do the same things like metal detecting and going to thrift stores. They both have a bit of a crazy streak that is identical and have the same sense of humor. My Gram always tells my dad to teach my brother and me what he knows. She says he has essential skills for life.

Back to a school for my future. My Gram worked in public schools for her entire career. She's seen the good, the bad, and the ugly. She is under no illusions about educators and what they can and cannot do. She can size a teacher or administrator up in seconds. Sometimes, it might be better to be oblivious to reality. Schools are overworked, underfunded, and, all too often, need to be more well-trained and resourced to deal with special needs students. We moved to a state where teachers don't seem to have a lot of respect, are paid horribly, and don't stay in teaching positions very long. She will not let me become a victim of that.

The Pillar of Parental Support

Imagine your parents as the almighty superheroes in your life, and you'll begin to understand the importance of their support when you have ADHD. They're like the Bat-Signal that shines brightly when you need guidance and assistance. Here's why parental consent is crucial for kids with ADHD.

Advocating for You

Parents are your first and most powerful advocates. They help you navigate the world, ensuring your needs are met at school, home, and other aspects of life. They're like your personal superheroes, standing up for you when it matters most.

Creating Structure

Consistency and routine are your trusty allies when you have ADHD. Parents provide the structure you need to thrive. They help establish daily schedules, organize your environment, and maintain a sense of predictability.

Medication Management

If you and your doctor decide medication is part of your ADHD management plan, parents must ensure you take it as prescribed. They keep track of your medication schedule and communicate with your healthcare team about any changes or concerns.

Emotional Support

Parents are your emotional anchors. They offer a safe space to express your feelings, whether frustrated, overwhelmed, or joyful. Their unconditional love and understanding provide comfort during challenging times.

Teaching Coping Strategies

Parents are your mentors, guiding you in developing coping strategies to manage ADHD-related challenges. They help you explore various techniques for staying organized, focused, and on track in school and daily life.

Encouragement and Positivity
Parents are your biggest cheerleaders. They celebrate your successes, no matter how small, and encourage you to believe in yourself. Their positive reinforcement boosts your self-esteem and confidence.

Fostering Independence
While offering support, parents also encourage your independence. They help you build essential life skills and decision-making abilities, empowering you to become a self-sufficient superhero.

Communication with Educators
Parents serve as your liaison with teachers and school administrators. They collaborate with educators to create an optimal learning environment, ensuring your unique needs are addressed in the classroom.

Resource Finding
Parents are expert treasure hunters. They seek out valuable resources, including books, support groups, and therapy options, to further assist you in managing your ADHD effectively.

Unconditional Love
Above all, parents provide unwavering love and acceptance. Their belief in your abilities, despite the challenges of ADHD, bolsters your self-worth and resilience.

In ADHD, parental support is like the unbreakable shield that helps you face challenges head-on and the guiding light that leads you to success. While having ADHD might make some tasks more challenging, with your parents' love and support, you have everything you need to conquer any obstacle that comes your way. Together, you make an unstoppable team!

54

Chapter 7

Doctor Visits

I want to share a little about going to the doctor to learn more about ADHD and get help. It can be scary at first, but it's essential to understand your brain to make it work better for you. When you have ADHD, those visits can be beneficial and reassuring. So, let's dive into what it's like when you're sitting in that cozy, but sometimes intimidating, doctor's office.

I've been on different medications since I was diagnosed in kindergarten. I haven't hit on one that works well for the entire day. My pediatrician diagnosed me at first, but then I was diagnosed by a clinical psychologist. The pediatrician has a daughter who has ADHD and has a learning disability, so she is very understanding. She knows the quirks of the ADHD brain. She also understands the limitations of the school system.

Before your visit the doctor, you, your parents, and your teacher might have to complete a questionnaire. It's a list of questions about your behavior, habits, and feelings. This helps the doctor understand you better.

Once you're in the doctor's office, you'll have a chat about your ADHD. It's like a conversation about your unique abilities. You can talk about the challenging things, like focusing in class or keeping your room organized. Sometimes, the doctor might ask you to do some tests or activities. It's not like being in school – there are no grades. These tests help determine how your brain works and what strategies might work best for you.

The Plan

After the chat and tests, you and the doctor will devise a plan. This plan might include strategies for school, like using a special fidget toy or trying out a new way to stay organized. If you are on medication, she will decide whether it needs to be adjusted. The doctor might also give you some tools to use daily. These tools can be like

55

gadgets. They might include a planner, apps, or meditation techniques to help you stay focused.

Medication

Now, let's talk about a topic that often arises when discussing ADHD: medication. I think of it as my trusty sidekick, working alongside me to help manage my ADHD.

There is a lot of information in the world on ADHD and medication. Some of it are myths, and some of it is true. This topic is emotional; people don't always know what to do. It can be unclear.

Medication for ADHD is like a tool. It's designed to help you manage some of the challenges that come with ADHD, especially regarding focus, attention, and impulse control. These medications work by adjusting the balance of certain chemicals in your brain to help you stay on track.

Types of Medication

There are two main types of medications for ADHD: stimulants and non-stimulants. Stimulants are the most commonly prescribed medications for ADHD. They might seem counterintuitive, but they work by calming the hyperactive parts of your brain, helping you focus better. Some examples include *Ritalin* and *Adderall*.

If stimulants don't work well for you, or you experience side effects, non-stimulant medications like *Strattera* might be an option. They work differently by affecting other brain chemicals.

Medication Superpowers

When a medication is the right fit, it can have some pretty cool superpowers of its own. It can:

Improve Focus

Medication can help you concentrate better, making it easier to pay attention in class, complete homework, and stay organized.

Reduced Impulsivity
It can help you think before you act, making it easier to resist the urge to yell out answers or interrupt others.

Calm the Storm
For some, medication can help reduce the whirlwind of thoughts and restlessness, creating a sense of calm.

Finding the Right Fit

Choosing whether to use medication for your ADHD is a big decision, and it's different for everyone. Some people find it extremely helpful, while others might prefer alternative strategies. Working closely with the doctor is essential to determine if the medication is proper.

Medication is just one part of the ADHD management team. It often works best with other strategies like therapy, lifestyle changes, and organizational techniques. Your family, teachers, and friends can also be part of your support network, helping you navigate your ADHD journey.

If you and your doctor decide to try medication, following the maker's instructions carefully is crucial. Regular check-ins will help ensure the medicine works as it should and you're not experiencing any unwanted side effects.

Remember, medication isn't a cure for ADHD, but it can be a powerful tool to help make life a little easier. The decision to use medication is highly individual, so have open and honest discussions with your doctor and family about what's best for you.

Chapter 8

Coping with Challenges

Life with ADHD isn't always easy, but there are ways to cope. I'll share some strategies for staying organized, managing emotions, and overcoming tough times. Let's get down to business and talk about how to cope with the unique challenges of inattentive type ADHD.

The Power of Planning
Planning is your trusty sidekick. Use tools like planners, calendars, or apps to keep track of assignments, deadlines, and important dates. Setting daily and weekly goals can help you stay on track and break down tasks into manageable chunks.

Organization is Key
Your secret lair (room, desk, or study space) should be tidy and well-organized. Invest in storage solutions, like shelves and bins, to keep your school materials in order. A clutter-free space can help declutter your mind.

Super Study Strategies
When studying, break your work into short, focused sessions. Use strategies like the *Pomodoro Technique*, which involves 25 minutes of intense work and a 5-minute break. This can help prevent boredom and improve your retention of information.

Mindful Listening
During class or conversations, practice active listening. Take notes, ask questions, and engage with the material. This can help you stay present and absorb information more effectively.

Fidget to Focus
Having a fidget toy or object to manipulate can help you stay attentive. It provides a way to channel excess energy and maintain focus without disruption.

Find Your Learning Style
Discover the way you learn best. Do you prefer visual aids, auditory cues, or hands-on experiences? Tailor your study methods to your learning style for more efficient learning.

Support System
Your friends, family, and teachers can be valuable allies. Feel free to communicate your needs to them. They can offer support and understanding when you're facing challenges.

Mindfulness and Meditation
Mindfulness techniques and meditation can help you center your thoughts and reduce distractions. These practices can improve your attention and overall well-being.

Break Tasks into Smaller Steps
When tackling large projects, divide them into smaller, more manageable tasks. It's easier to focus on one step at a time, and the sense of accomplishment as you complete each step can be motivating.

Reward Yourself
Remember to celebrate your victories, no matter how small. Give yourself rewards, like a favorite snack or a short break, to acknowledge your efforts and maintain motivation.

Exercise and Diet
Physical activity can help burn off excess energy and improve focus. Likewise, a balanced diet can positively impact attention and overall well-being.

Seek Professional Help

If ADHD continues to impact your life significantly, consider seeking professional help. Therapy, such as cognitive-behavioral therapy (CBT), can provide valuable strategies and coping skills.

Remember, you're unique with your own set of tools and talents. What works best for you might be different from what works for others. Be patient, keep experimenting with these coping strategies, and don't forget you're not alone on this ADHD adventure.

You've got a whole team of supporters, friends, family, and yourself working together to make each day brighter and more successful.

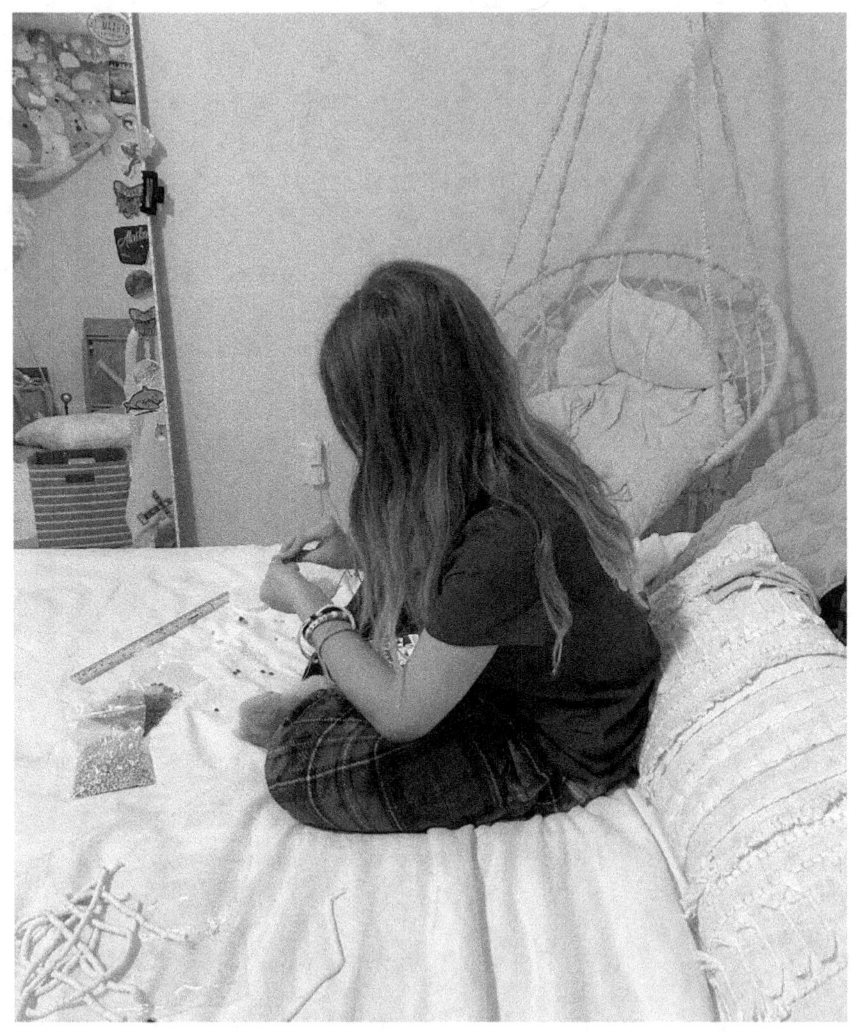

I am going to be honest. My parents help me with most of this stuff. Sometimes, I can do it quickly; other times, I struggle. Now that we've moved to a different area, my mom is investigating psychiatrists specializing in ADHD. I don't think I need therapy; I think I need the proper medication.

Chapter 9

Navigating Hostile or Poorly Informed Educators

Sometimes, educators need help understanding you or don't want to make the necessary accommodations. I only ran into this once, but that incident took up almost a year. This is a tricky subject for me because I have, for the most part, loved my teachers. I respect teachers, and most of them are lovely. However, I've dealt with educators who don't understand ADHD, don't want to understand ADHD, and are hostile to my mom's advocacy for me.

As mentioned, my Gram does not look at the school system through rose-colored glasses. In your journey with ADHD, you'll encounter many understanding and supportive educators. Still, there may be times when you come across educators who are less receptive to suggestions for helping ADHD kids. Here's how to navigate those situations and how parents can advocate effectively for the support you need.

Stay Calm and Patient
When facing resistance, it's essential to remain calm and patient. Remember that some educators may not have much experience with ADHD or might not fully understand it. Give them time to learn and adapt.

Educate and Share Information
Provide educators with information about ADHD. Share reputable articles, books, or resources that explain the condition and its impact on learning. Knowledge is often the first step toward empathy and support.

Build a Positive Relationship
Work on building a positive and respectful relationship with the educator. Open lines of communication and demonstrate

your willingness to collaborate for the benefit of the child with ADHD.

Use "I" Statements

Use "I" statements to express your feelings and needs when discussing concerns or suggestions. For example, say, "I have noticed that my child benefits from shorter, more frequent breaks," rather than making accusatory statements.

Focus on the Child's Needs

Emphasize that your suggestions are based on what you believe will best meet the child's educational and developmental needs. Highlight how the suggested accommodations can help the child succeed.

Offer Practical Solutions

Present concrete, practical solutions that the educator can implement in the classroom. Be specific about the accommodations or strategies you suggest and how they can be integrated into the curriculum.

Request a Meeting

If you're facing resistance, request a meeting with the educator and possibly other school staff, such as a school counselor or special education coordinator. A face-to-face conversation can often lead to a better understanding of the child's needs.

Collaborate with Experts

If necessary, involve professionals specializing in ADHD, such as a school psychologist or educational consultant. Their expertise can help address any concerns and provide additional insights.

Document Conversations

Keep records of your interactions with educators. Note the conversations' date, time, content, and any agreements or action plans. This documentation can be valuable if you need to escalate the issue.

Seek Higher Levels of Support

If efforts to work with the educator are unsuccessful, you can escalate the issue to higher levels of school administration or the school district. Be prepared to advocate for your child's rights under the Individuals with Disabilities Education Act (IDEA) or Section 504 of the Rehabilitation Act if applicable.

Join Support Groups

Connect with other parents who have children with ADHD. They can offer advice, support, and guidance based on their experiences with educators and schools.

Stay Persistent

Advocating for a child with ADHD can sometimes be a lengthy process. Don't give up. Continue to advocate persistently for your child's support to thrive in the educational environment.

Remember that the goal is to create an environment where children with ADHD can learn and grow to their fullest potential. While encountering hostile educators can be challenging, your advocacy efforts can make a significant difference in ensuring that the children's needs are met and they receive the support they deserve.

One of the most challenging situations for a parent and a student is uninformed educators who think they know it all and resent spending time making accommodations for you. They may not believe that ADHD is real. I think these people are, by far, in the minority, but this is a huge issue when it happens, and I wanted to talk a little about it.

504 Plan

Remember I told you that I had a 504 plan? Well, that plan lays out accommodations for me to be successful in school. The 504 plan is reviewed yearly, or whenever the school or parent asks to be reviewed. I have accommodations like needing extra time to take tests and needing to be retaught math concepts missed on tests and retested.

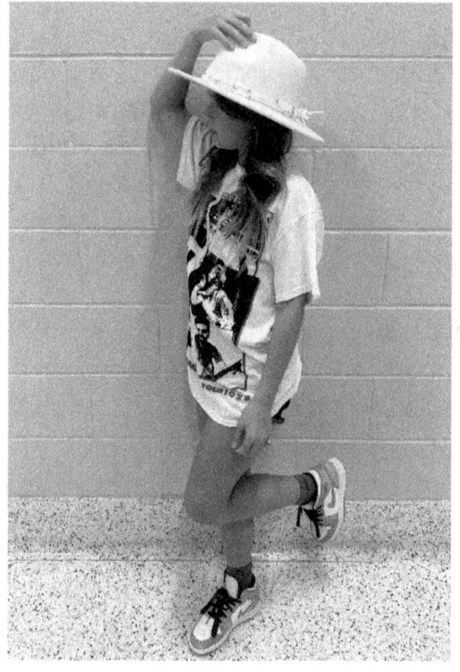

I don't want to go into the law right now, but if you are going to advocate for yourself, or if your parents are going to be your advocates, you have to know your rights. Because not all teachers or administrators know this information, and it can hurt you.

This happened when my mom asked for an accommodation for me in math. The school's assistant principal told her that, "It wouldn't be fair to the other students," and "What would the parents of the other students think?" I don't think this is legal. The assistant principal should've known better. I was refused an accommodation all year that could have helped me.

It hurts a lot when people who should know better say careless and what I think are illegal things. When educators don't know the law or understand the rights of a disabled child, they do her a real disservice and demoralize her. My mom could have stepped back, but she fought for me. Unfortunately, the principal was also very poorly informed and didn't understand what ADHD is all about.

A 504 plan, also known as a Section 504 plan, is a legally binding document in the United States that outlines accommodations and support services for students with disabilities. It is named after Section 504 of the Rehabilitation Act of 1973, a federal law prohibiting discrimination against individuals with disabilities in programs and activities receiving federal financial assistance, including public schools.

A 504 plan ensures that students with disabilities have equal access to education and the opportunity to participate in school programs and activities. While it doesn't provide individualized instruction like an Individualized Education Program (IEP), it does outline specific accommodations and modifications that can help a student with a disability succeed in a general education setting. Here are some critical components of a 504 plan.

Eligibility
To qualify for a 504 plan, a student must have a physical or mental impairment substantially limiting one or more major life activities. Major life activities include walking, seeing, hearing, learning, concentrating, and interacting with others. ADHD and other conditions, including medical conditions, may qualify a student for a 504 plan.

Evaluation
The school determines if the student meets the eligibility criteria. This evaluation may include input from teachers, parents, and other professionals.

Accommodations and Services
If a student is found eligible, a 504 plan is developed. This plan outlines specific accommodations, services, and modifications that the student will receive. Examples of accommodations for students with ADHD may include extended time on tests, preferential seating, access to a quiet space for focus, and using organizational tools.

Implementation
Teachers and school staff are responsible for implementing the accommodations and services outlined in the 504 plan. Regular communication between parents, teachers, and other relevant school personnel is essential to ensure the plan's effectiveness.

Periodic Review

504 plans are typically reviewed periodically to assess the student's progress and make any necessary adjustments to accommodations. Parents, teachers, and the student (when appropriate) should participate in these reviews.

Parental Rights
Parents have the right to be involved in developing and reviewing the 504 plan. They also have the right to request an evaluation or appeal decisions related to the plan.

Confidentiality
Information related to a student's 504 plan is confidential and should only be shared with individuals who need to know.

It's important to note that while a 504 plan can provide valuable support for students with disabilities, it is not the same as an IEP. IEPs offer more extensive and individualized services, including specialized instruction, and are typically reserved for students with more significant disabilities.

If you believe you may benefit from a 504 plan, it is recommended that you contact the special education or 504 coordinator to initiate the evaluation process. They can guide eligibility and develop a plan tailored to your child's needs.

We moved over the summer, and my new school called for a 504 plan review. My latest math teacher said she provided a unique accommodation that should be in my plan. Without being asked, she was doing what my old school had denied!

Chapter 10

Taking the Dreaded Computerized State Standardized Tests

Taking computerized state standardized tests can be challenging for students, especially those with ADHD. These tests, which have become increasingly common in educational systems, present unique student difficulties and stressors. Here are some reasons why computerized state standardized tests can be challenging.

Sensory Overload
Some students with ADHD are sensitive to sensory stimuli, including the bright screens, sounds, and headphones or earbuds required during computerized tests. These sensory elements can overwhelm and distract them.

Attention and Focus
Students with ADHD often struggle with maintaining sustained attention and focus. Computerized tests require continuous attention for extended periods and can exacerbate these challenges.

Time Management
Managing time during computerized tests can be complex for students with ADHD, as they may struggle with pacing themselves effectively to complete all sections within the allotted time.

Impulsivity
Impulsivity is a common symptom of ADHD. On computerized tests, impulsivity may lead to hasty, inaccurate responses rather than thoughtful and accurate answers.

Technical Issues

Technical glitches, such as freezing screens, crashes, or slow response times, can create stress and disrupt the testing experience. This can be particularly frustrating for students with ADHD, who may already find the testing environment overwhelming.

Anxiety and Pressure
The high-stakes nature of state standardized tests can lead to stress, and for students with ADHD, this anxiety can be more pronounced due to the fear of not completing the quiz or making mistakes.

Limited Breaks
Some computerized tests offer little or no breaks between sections, which can be challenging for students with ADHD who may need short breaks to recharge and refocus.

Incompatibility with Accommodations
Some students with ADHD require accommodations such as extended time, preferential seating, or paper-and-pencil tests. Computerized tests may only sometimes be compatible with these accommodations.

Lack of Personalization
Computerized tests often need more personalization and flexibility than traditional paper tests. This can be less accommodating for students with ADHD, who may benefit from adjustments based on their individual needs.

One-Size-Fits-All Doesn't Work
To address these challenges, educators and schools must consider the unique needs of students with ADHD during standardized testing. This may include providing accommodations, such as extended time, offering quiet and distraction-free testing environments, and incorporating regular short breaks. Additionally, teaching students with ADHD test-taking strategies, self-regulation

techniques, and mindfulness exercises can help them better manage their symptoms during computerized tests.

A one-size-fits-all standardized test does not work well for disabled kids, including those with conditions like ADHD, because it fails to account for these students' diverse learning needs, abilities, and challenges. Here are several vital reasons why standardized tests often fall short for disabled children.

Diverse Disabilities

Disabled children encompass various conditions, each with unique characteristics and impacts on learning. ADHD, autism, dyslexia, and physical disabilities affect students differently. A single standardized test cannot accurately assess their varying abilities and challenges.

Variability in Cognitive Functioning

Children with disabilities may have cognitive functioning outside the norm. Some may excel in certain areas while struggling in others. Standardized tests typically do not allow this variation in cognitive strengths and weaknesses.

Accommodation Needs

Many disabled children require accommodations, such as extended time, use of assistive technology, or alternative formats (e.g., large print or braille), to access and complete assessments effectively. One-size-fits-all tests often do not provide these necessary accommodations.

Inequitable Testing Conditions

The standardized testing environment may not accommodate the sensory sensitivities, attention deficits, or physical limitations of disabled students. This can lead to increased stress and test anxiety, negatively impacting performance.

Communication Barriers

For children with communication disorders or speech impairments, standardized tests relying heavily on written or spoken responses may not accurately reflect their knowledge and abilities.

Emotional and Psychological Factors

Many disabled students face emotional and psychological challenges related to their disabilities. The stress and pressure associated with standardized testing can exacerbate these issues and affect test performance.

Underrepresentation

Some standardized tests have been criticized for underrepresenting certain disabilities or not including specific accommodations, disadvantaging children with less common conditions.

Stigmatization

Standardized tests can contribute to the stigmatization of disabled students. When their performance on these tests is used to make comparisons or judgments, it can reinforce negative stereotypes and impact their self-esteem.

Narrow Assessment of Abilities

Standardized tests typically focus on limited skills and knowledge, emphasizing rote memorization and regurgitation of facts. They may not effectively measure the broader skills, creativity, problem-solving abilities, and talents of disabled students.

Limited Validity

The validity of standardized tests for disabled children may be questioned, as they may not accurately capture the true extent of a student's knowledge or abilities.

A Flexible Approach

Given these challenges, it's essential to recognize the need for more inclusive and flexible assessment approaches that account for the individualized needs of disabled children. This may involve:

Tailored Assessments
Developing assessments that align with the specific needs and abilities of disabled students, allowing for accommodations and alternative response formats.

Alternative Assessments
Considering alternative assessment methods, such as performance-based tasks, portfolios, or teacher observations, provides a more comprehensive view of a student's abilities.

Emphasis on Growth
Shifting the focus from comparing students to measuring their individual growth and progress over time is a more equitable way to assess their development.

Incorporating Teacher Input
Recognizing the valuable insights of teachers and specialists who work closely with disabled students and involving them in the assessment process.

Advocating for Inclusivity
Advocating for policies and practices prioritizing inclusive education, individualized accommodations, and support services to ensure disabled students have an equal opportunity to succeed.

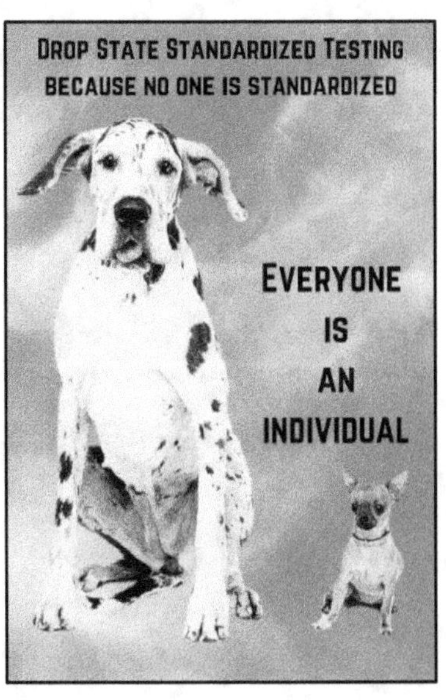

My state spends about $54.3 million each year on testing. I may be just a kid, but I think I could find a better way to provide kids with what they need than sitting in front of a computer screen.

Standardized tests, when used without consideration for the diverse needs of disabled children, can be an inadequate and inequitable measure of their abilities. A more inclusive and personalized approach to assessment is essential to ensure that all students, regardless of their disabilities, are given a fair and accurate opportunity to demonstrate their knowledge and skills.

Chapter 11

Shame

ADHD inattentive type can lead to feelings of shame in girls for several reasons. Understanding why they experience this shame and how to address it is crucial for their emotional well-being and self-esteem.

I don't know if shame is a good descriptor for me. Maybe sometimes. It isn't easy to have everyone else understand while I sit there. It seems like I always need extra help. That can be very uncomfortable. No one, not teachers, peers, or family, makes me feel ashamed. I think it is something in all of us. We feel it when we aren't in sync with everyone else.

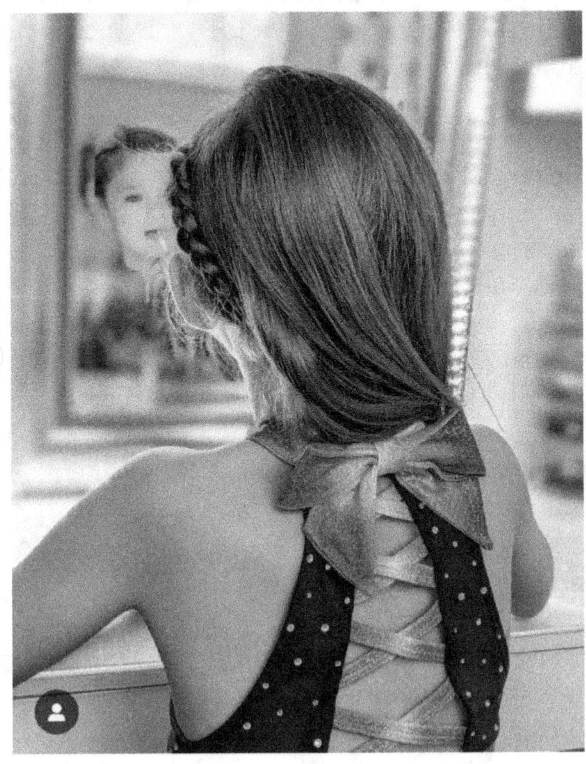

Why Girls with ADHD Feel Shame:

Perceived Differences
Girls with ADHD inattentive type often notice their differences in attention, organization, and focus compared to their peers. These differences can make them feel like they don't fit in or that something is wrong with them.

Academic Struggles
ADHD can lead to academic challenges, such as forgetfulness, difficulty completing assignments, or lower grades. These struggles can erode self-confidence and lead to feelings of incompetence.

Social Comparisons
Girls may compare themselves to friends who seem more organized or academically successful. This can intensify feelings of inadequacy, as they may perceive themselves as falling short.

Stigma and Misunderstanding
There is still a stigma surrounding ADHD, and girls with the inattentive type may face misconceptions about their condition. This can lead to feelings of shame, as they fear being judged or misunderstood.

Internalized Messages
Girls with ADHD may internalize negative messages from others or societal expectations about how they should perform academically or behaviorally. These internalized beliefs can contribute to shame.

Addressing Shame in Girls with ADHD

Education and Understanding
Provide age-appropriate information about ADHD to help girls understand their condition better. Knowledge can reduce

stigma and help them recognize that ADHD is not a personal failure.

Open Communication

Create an open and nonjudgmental environment where girls feel comfortable discussing their feelings and challenges related to ADHD. Please encourage them to express their emotions.

Emphasize Strengths

Focus on and celebrate their strengths, talents, and achievements. Help them recognize that ADHD does not define their worth or potential.

Normalize Differences

Normalize the idea that everyone has unique strengths and challenges. Explain that having ADHD is just one aspect of who they are.

Set Realistic Expectations

Work with them to set realistic goals and expectations for their academic and personal lives. Help them understand that it's okay to ask for help when needed.

Teach Coping Strategies

Teach practical coping strategies for managing ADHD symptoms. This can include techniques for organization, time management, and focus.

Seek Professional Help

Consider involving mental health professionals or educational specialists who can provide guidance, strategies, and support tailored to their needs.

Build Self-Esteem
Encourage activities and hobbies that boost their self-esteem and self-worth. Participation in extracurricular activities or pursuits they enjoy can foster a sense of achievement.

Advocate for Accommodations
If needed, advocate for educational accommodations and support at school. These can help level the playing field and reduce the academic pressure contributing to shame.

Emphasize Resilience
Teach them that resilience is a valuable trait. Share stories of successful individuals who have overcome ADHD-related challenges.

Peer Support
Encourage girls to connect with peers who have similar experiences. Support groups or friendships with others who understand ADHD can reduce feelings of isolation.

Patience and Self-Compassion
Teach them the importance of patience with themselves and self-compassion. Remind them that mistakes and setbacks are part of the learning process.

Addressing shame related to ADHD inattentive type is an ongoing process. It's essential to provide consistent support, encouragement, and a safe space for girls to express their feelings and seek help when needed. By fostering a positive self-image and resilience, girls with ADHD can develop the confidence to navigate challenges and embrace their unique strengths.

I want to return to the computerized state testing discussed in the last chapter. I consistently get a level 1 in math. That is the lowest score you can get on these automated state tests. That can bring shame, and it can also bring a sense of hopelessness. Why try?

Chapter 12

Technology and ADHD

Several types of assistive technology and software tools can benefit girls with ADHD inattentive type. These tools enhance organization, time management, focus, and productivity. Here are some examples.

Digital Calendars and Reminder Apps
Google Calendar, Apple Calendar, or *Microsoft Outlook*: These digital calendar apps allow users to schedule events, set reminders, and organize their daily activities. They can help girls with ADHD keep track of assignments, appointments, and deadlines.

Task Management Apps
Todoist, Trello, or *Asana*: Task management apps enable users to create to-do lists, set priorities, and track progress on assignments and projects. They can help girls with ADHD stay organized and break tasks into manageable steps.

Note-Taking Apps
Evernote, OneNote, or *Notion*: These note-taking apps provide a digital platform for capturing and organizing notes, ideas, and research materials. They often include features for categorizing information and searching for keywords.

Text-to-Speech and Speech-to-Text Software
Read&Write, Dragon NaturallySpeaking, or *Google's Voice Typing*: These tools assist with reading and writing tasks. Text-to-speech software reads text aloud, while speech-to-text software converts spoken words into text. They can help girls with ADHD process information and express their thoughts more efficiently.

Focus and Time Management Tools

StayFocusd, Freedom, or *Cold Turkey*: These apps allow users to block distracting websites and apps, set time limits for online activities, and improve their focus during study sessions.

Mindfulness and Relaxation Apps

Calm, Headspace, or *Insight Timer*: Mindfulness apps offer guided meditation sessions and relaxation exercises to help girls with ADHD manage stress, reduce anxiety, and improve attention.

Reading Assistance Tools

Kurzweil 3000 or *NaturalReader*: These tools can assist with reading comprehension by highlighting text as it is read aloud. They also offer customizable settings for font size, color, and background.

Graphic Organizers and Mind Mapping Software

MindMeister, XMind, or *Lucidspark*: These tools support visual thinking and brainstorming. They can help girls with ADHD organize ideas, create outlines, and visualize relationships between concepts.

Digital Flashcards

Quizlet, Anki, or *Brainscape*: Flashcard apps allow users to create digital flashcards for studying. They often include features like spaced repetition to enhance memory retention.

Focus-Enhancing Wearables

Devices like smartwatches and fitness trackers can include features that remind users to take breaks, stay active, and maintain healthy sleep patterns.

Customizable Keyboard Shortcuts and Macros
Customizing keyboard shortcuts and macros on a computer can save time and effort for those who struggle with keyboard navigation and repetitive tasks.

Noise-Canceling Headphones
Noise-canceling headphones can create a quieter study environment, reducing distractions for girls with ADHD.

When selecting assistive technology tools, it's essential to consider the specific needs and preferences of the individual. Some devices may be more effective than others, so it may require trial and error to find the right combination of assistive technology that works best for a girl with ADHD inattentive type. Additionally, involving teachers, parents, or professionals who specialize in ADHD support can provide valuable insights and recommendations for choosing and implementing these tools effectively.

Chapter 13

Celebrating Successes

Having ADHD means I can do amazing things. I'll tell you about some of my proudest moments and how I celebrate my successes. As I've mentioned, I play ice hockey. I live and breathe ice hockey.

Because my family moved from one part of our state to another this past summer, I wasn't sure what would happen with my hockey career. I had just made an elite girl's hockey team when we left. I was sad and happy. I guess you call that mixed emotions. I didn't want to leave my friends and new group, but I'd been part of finding a new home and was excited about where we planned to move.

My mom and dad found a new ice rink with teams. The traveling or elite teams had already been chosen, but the tryouts for the rec teams had yet to be. My mom signed me up for rec.

As I was skating on the first night of practice, the coach approached my mom and said, "Who is this girl? I know every female ice hockey skater in the area, and I have never seen her." My mom explained about the move. He told her he was also the traveling team's coach and wanted me on that team!!!! It was the 12 and under team!!!!! I was so excited I couldn't sleep that night. He thought I was terrific. Wow!

I'm now on the rec team, which ends in December, and the traveling team, which ends in the spring. On my traveling team, we will travel all over my state and some new states I've never been to.

Part of the traveling team's practice includes meeting with a Life Coach monthly. The Life Coach teaches us how to keep calm and focused. How to deal with bullies and overly aggressive players positively and manage emotions. Is this perfect for a kid with ADHD, or what?

My mom is candid about my condition and ensures all my teachers and coaches understand that I have ADHD. She pulled my coach aside at our second practice and told him, and guess what he said! "I have ADHD too. I process differently than others, and sometimes people misread me. I talk to myself to help me understand, and the refs will ask me if I question their calls."

Oh, my goodness! An adult who understands because he rides the ADHD roller coaster, too!

My mom told him that I'm never a behavior problem or disrespectful, but I can look like I'm not listening, but I am. He said that's precisely how he is, too! He gets it! That's like being given a wonderful gift. That's a whole celebration. I was hand-picked for the traveling team and have a coach who understands me!

More Reasons to Celebrate

Another celebration for me is my friendships. I've talked about that. My former teacher told my mom I got the most votes when she asked everyone who they wanted to sit with. My new teacher said I was in a lovely peer group. The good thing about friendships is that you can be part of them daily, and they can occur in school and out.

I hope to get to know my new hockey teammates. It's still early to get a friendship going, but I'm confident I'll succeed. I'm very tech-savvy, and my friends and I take advantage of communicating via our iPhones.

My looks are another reason to celebrate. I'm cautious of my appearance. I've learned to put on light makeup and wear a little jewelry that isn't over the top. I have a very low-key style…usually! My old school had a dance last year and I wore a dress and my Jordan high tops.

I did some modeling in Cheer and traveled to a few cities outside our state to participate in shoots. I loved it. I made friends and connected with some charming people. I want to continue modeling so I can continue traveling and meeting people. This isn't politically correct, but I want to celebrate my looks. I want to know that I am above average at a few things. I know that looks fade, but I figure I have some time.

Chapter 14

Coping Strategies and Caring for a Pet

There's an arsenal of coping strategies at my disposal. From using organizational tools to mindfulness techniques. I can build a toolkit tailored to my needs. I experiment with various methods to discover what works best for me.

Navigating life with inattentive type ADHD sometimes feels like a challenging quest, but with the right strategies, I can harness my unique strengths and thrive. Here are some tailored coping strategies that I think apply to me and other kids with inattentive type ADHD.

Organize
Use color coding for notebooks, folders, and calendars to help keep track of assignments and due dates. Invest in a planner or digital calendar to record tasks, appointments, and important dates.

Chunk: Break Tasks into Bite-Sized Pieces
When faced with a daunting task, break it down into smaller, more manageable steps. Create a checklist to track progress. Use timers or alarms to stay on track and allocate specific time blocks for different tasks.

Minimize Distractions
Find a quiet and clutter-free study space to focus without interruptions. Use noise-canceling headphones or soft background music to create a conducive environment for concentration.

Prioritize Self-Care
Get enough sleep, eat nutritious meals, and engage in regular physical activity. A healthy body supports a healthy mind.

Practice mindfulness, deep breathing, or yoga to help manage stress and anxiety.

Utilize Technology

Explore apps and digital tools to help with organization, time management, and task tracking. Use voice memos or speech-to-text apps for capturing ideas or taking notes when writing feels overwhelming.

Leverage Creativity

Embrace creativity and use it as an advantage. Incorporate art, visualization, or creative projects into the learning process. Create mnemonic devices or visual aids to remember information more effectively.

Stay Connected

Maintain open communication with family, friends, and teachers. They can provide support and assistance when needed. Consider joining support groups or online communities for girls with ADHD to connect with others with similar experiences.

Celebrate Achievements

Acknowledge and celebrate successes, no matter how small. Positive reinforcement can boost self-esteem and motivation. Please don't dwell on setbacks; view them as learning opportunities and growth.

Learn and Practice Self Advocacy

Develop self-advocacy skills. Learn to express needs and preferences to teachers, parents, and peers. Feel free to ask for accommodations or adjustments in the classroom to help you learn more effectively.

Seek Professional Guidance

Consider working with a therapist or counselor who specializes in ADHD. They can provide valuable strategies and emotional support. If medication is part of a treatment plan, follow the doctor's recommendations carefully and communicate any concerns or side effects.

ADHD Doesn't Define You

Remember, ADHD is just one facet of an identity. Embrace strengths, persevere through challenges, and continue to learn and grow. With determination and the right strategies, the world can be navigated well.

ADHD doesn't define you; it's just one aspect of who you are. Explore your passions, discover your interests, and enthusiastically pursue your dreams. Your unique perspective can lead to extraordinary achievements.

It's essential to convey that ADHD is just one aspect of me and doesn't define my entire identity. Here's why ADHD doesn't interpret my life for me.

I'm Multifaceted

I have many interests, talents, and personality traits beyond ADHD. I'm not just someone with a neurodevelopmental disorder; I'm a unique individual with strengths and weaknesses.

ADHD is a Part of Me, Not All of Me

While ADHD impacts certain aspects of my life, it doesn't define my worth or potential. It's one facet of my identity, similar to other traits like my sense of humor, creativity, or kindness.

I'm More than My Challenges

ADHD comes with challenges, such as difficulty with focus and organization, but it doesn't overshadow my abilities. I have talents, skills, and accomplishments that I'm proud of and that showcase my capabilities.

I'm Resilient

Dealing with ADHD has made me resilient and adaptable. I've learned strategies to manage my symptoms and continue to grow and develop. My ability to overcome challenges is a significant part of who I am.

ADHD Can Be an Asset

ADHD isn't just a list of deficits. It can be an asset too. It often brings creativity, energy, and a unique perspective. I've learned to harness these qualities to my advantage.

I'm Still Learning and Growing

I'm on a journey of self-discovery and personal growth, just like anyone else. ADHD is part of that journey, but doesn't limit my growth, learning, and self-improvement potential.

I Have Dreams and Goals

I have dreams, aspirations, and goals I'm passionate about. My ADHD may pose challenges along the way, but it doesn't deter me from pursuing my ambitions and striving for success.

I'm Part of a Diverse Community

Many people, including some of my friends and peers, also have ADHD. It's comforting to know I'm not alone in my experiences and can learn from and support others within the ADHD community.

I Define Myself

Ultimately, I am the one who defines who I am, not a diagnosis. I choose how I perceive myself and navigate the world, including how I address and manage ADHD.

I'm Loved and Supported

My family, friends, and support network love and accept me for who I am. They see beyond my diagnosis and appreciate the unique qualities that make me who I am.

ADHD is a part of my life but doesn't encompass my entire being. I am a multifaceted individual with a wealth of experiences, talents, and dreams that go beyond the challenges posed by ADHD. I define myself and focus on my strengths and aspirations as I grow and thrive.

Be Honest

Being honest about your ADHD and being able to explain it to others is a crucial aspect of self-advocacy and fostering understanding in your personal and professional relationships. Here's why it's important and some tips on how to do it effectively.

The Importance of Honesty and Explanation

Self-Acceptance

Being open about your ADHD allows you to embrace and accept it as part of your identity. Acceptance is the first step toward effectively managing and thriving with ADHD.

Reducing Stigma

Open and honest conversations about ADHD can help reduce the stigma associated with the condition. By sharing your experiences, you contribute to greater awareness and understanding.

Practical Support

When you explain your ADHD to others, especially in a personal or school context, it helps them understand your unique needs and challenges. This can lead to more effective support and accommodations.

Improved Relationships

Being honest about your ADHD fosters trust and authenticity in your relationships. It allows others to see the real you, including your strengths and vulnerabilities.

Tips for Explaining Your ADHD

Educate Yourself
Before explaining ADHD to others, understand the condition well. This includes its symptoms, how it affects you personally, and any strategies or treatments you use.

Choose the Right Time and Place
Pick an appropriate setting for your conversation where you and the other person can focus and have a private, uninterrupted discussion.

Be Clear and Concise
Keep your explanation simple and to the point. Describe ADHD in a way that someone unfamiliar with the condition can understand. You might say, "ADHD is a neurodevelopmental disorder that affects my attention, focus, and sometimes my impulse control."

Share Personal Experiences
Use real-life examples to illustrate how ADHD manifests daily. Sharing personal anecdotes can make the condition more relatable.

Discuss Coping Strategies
Explain your strategies and techniques to manage your ADHD. This could include medication, therapy, organization tools, or time-management methods.

Express Your Needs
Be clear about the support or accommodations you require. Letting others know your needs is essential, whether it's a quiet workspace, flexible deadlines, or specific communication styles.

Emphasize Strengths

Highlight your strengths and talents. ADHD often comes with unique qualities like creativity, hyper-focus, and adaptability. Emphasizing these positives can balance the conversation.

Answer Questions

Be open to questions and provide factual, non-judgmental answers. People may have misconceptions about ADHD, so your willingness to clarify can be enlightening.

Practice Active Listening

Encourage the other person to share their thoughts and concerns. Active listening can lead to a more constructive and empathetic dialogue.

Patience and Understanding

Recognize that some people may need time to process and adjust to this new information. Be patient and understanding as they learn more about your ADHD.

Being honest about your ADHD and explaining it to others is a powerful way to foster understanding and support in your personal and professional relationships. It's a process of self-advocacy that can lead to more inclusive and empathetic interactions, ultimately benefiting you and those around you.

Caring for Pets

A pet can benefit children with ADHD. While pets may not replace professional treatment or interventions, they can play a valuable role in supporting the well-being of children with ADHD. Here's how having a pet can help.

Companionship and Emotional Support

Pets like dogs or cats offer constant companionship and emotional support. For children with ADHD, who may sometimes struggle with social interactions, a pet can provide a reliable source of comfort and friendship.

Routine and Responsibility

Caring for a pet involves establishing feeding, grooming, and exercise routines. This can help children with ADHD develop essential skills in time management, organization, and responsibility.

Physical Activity and Exercise

Many pets, especially dogs, require regular exercise. Engaging in physical activities like playing fetch or taking walks with a pet can help children with ADHD burn off excess energy and improve their focus and impulse control.

Stress Reduction

Interacting with pets has been shown to reduce stress and anxiety. This can be particularly beneficial for children with ADHD, who may experience heightened stress levels due to their condition or academic pressures.

Sensory Stimulation

The sensory experience of petting a soft animal, hearing their purring or breathing, and feeling their warmth can be soothing for children with ADHD, helping them relax and reduce sensory overload.

Improved Mood and Emotional Regulation

Spending time with a beloved pet can trigger the release of feel-good hormones like oxytocin and serotonin. This can improve mood and emotional regulation, reducing the likelihood of emotional outbursts.

Enhanced Social Skills

Interacting with a pet can improve a child's social skills, such as empathy, communication, and non-verbal cues. These skills can then transfer to interactions with peers and adults.

Unconditional Love and Acceptance

Pets offer unconditional love and acceptance. Children with ADHD may sometimes struggle with self-esteem or feelings of inadequacy. The love and non-judgmental companionship of a pet can boost their self-worth.

Learning Opportunities

Having a pet provides opportunities for learning about biology, animal behavior, and caregiving. Children with ADHD can engage in educational activities related to their pet's needs and well-being.

Reduced Feelings of Isolation

Children with ADHD may sometimes feel isolated or misunderstood. A pet can serve as a loyal and non-judgmental confidant, reducing feelings of loneliness.

Teaching Empathy and Responsibility

Caring for a pet teaches children the importance of empathy, compassion, and responsibility. These lessons can be valuable as they develop interpersonal skills.

It's important to note that the choice of a pet should align with the family's lifestyle, preferences, and the child's specific needs. Additionally, parents should take the primary responsibility for the pet's care while involving the child in age-appropriate tasks to ensure both the child's and the pet's well-being.

While pets can be wonderful companions for children with ADHD, they are not a substitute for professional medical or therapeutic interventions when needed. Parents should consult healthcare professionals and educators to create a comprehensive plan supporting their child's needs.

Chapter 15

Exercise and ADHD

Exercise can be a valuable and practical component of managing ADHD symptoms. It offers a range of physical, cognitive, and emotional benefits that can help individuals with ADHD improve focus, impulse control, and overall well-being. Here's how exercise can positively impact individuals with ADHD:

Increased Neurotransmitters

Exercise stimulates the release of neurotransmitters like dopamine and norepinephrine. These brain chemicals are crucial in regulating attention, mood, and motivation, often affecting individuals with ADHD.

Enhanced Cognitive Functioning

Regular physical activity can enhance cognitive functions, including attention and working memory. This can help individuals with ADHD focus more on tasks and reduce distractibility.

Reduced Hyperactivity and Impulsivity

Exercise can help channel excess energy and reduce hyperactivity and impulsivity. Engaging in physical activities can provide an outlet for restless energy and promote self-control.

Enhanced Executive Functioning

Exercise has been shown to improve executive functioning skills such as planning, organization, and time management, often impaired in individuals with ADHD.

Stress Reduction
Exercise is a natural stress reliever. It can reduce anxiety and help individuals with ADHD manage emotional fluctuations, improving overall mood.

Better Sleep
Regular physical activity can enhance sleep quality and regulate sleep patterns. Improved sleep can increase alertness and better cognitive functioning during the day.

Self-Esteem and Confidence
Achieving physical fitness goals can boost self-esteem and confidence, which may be particularly important for individuals with ADHD who struggle with self-doubt.

Social Interaction
Participating in team sports or group fitness activities can provide opportunities for social interaction and developing interpersonal skills.

Routine and Structure
Incorporating exercise into a daily routine can help individuals with ADHD establish structure and consistency in their lives, making managing daily tasks and responsibilities more manageable.

Long-Term Health Benefits
Regular physical activity is associated with improved cardiovascular health, reduced risk of obesity, and better overall physical health. These benefits contribute to an individual's long-term well-being.

It's important to note that the type and intensity of exercise can vary from person to person. Some individuals prefer team sports, while others like solitary activities like jogging or swimming. The key is to find an exercise routine that is enjoyable and sustainable. Ice hockey is enjoyable and sustainable to me. It's a team sport but, has a little solitary component.

Chapter 16

A Balanced Diet and ADHD

I'll be honest with you. I love junk food, processed foods, and sugar. I'm improving at eating a more balanced diet, but it can be challenging. Eating a balanced and nutritious diet can positively impact managing inattentive type ADHD symptoms. While diet alone isn't a substitute for other treatments and strategies, it can complement them and contribute to overall well-being. Here are dietary recommendations for individuals with ADHD:

Balanced Meals
Ensure that your meals are balanced, including various nutrient-rich foods from different food groups. Aim for lean proteins, whole grains, fruits, vegetables, and healthy fats.

Protein-Rich Foods
Include high-quality protein sources, such as lean meats, poultry, fish, beans, lentils, tofu, and dairy products. Protein can help stabilize blood sugar levels and improve focus.

Omega-3 Fatty Acids
Omega-3 fatty acids in fatty fish (e.g., salmon, mackerel), flaxseeds, and walnuts support brain health and cognitive function. Consider incorporating these foods into your diet.

Complex Carbohydrates
Opt for complex carbohydrates like whole grains (brown rice, whole wheat bread, quinoa) and legumes. These provide a steady release of energy and help maintain stable blood sugar levels.

Avoid Sugar and Processed Foods

Minimize or eliminate sugary snacks and processed foods from your diet. These can lead to energy spikes and crashes, affecting focus and attention.

Regular Meals and Snacks

Maintain a regular eating schedule, including balanced meals and nutritious snacks between meals. Consistent eating patterns can help stabilize mood and energy levels.

Hydration

Stay well-hydrated by drinking plenty of water throughout the day. Dehydration can lead to fatigue and decreased cognitive function.

Limit Food Additives

Some individuals with ADHD may be sensitive to certain food additives, such as artificial colors and preservatives. Consider reducing or avoiding foods and drinks with these additives.

Iron and Zinc

Ensure an adequate iron and zinc intake through lean meats, poultry, beans, nuts, and fortified cereals. These minerals are essential for cognitive function.

Vitamin D

Adequate vitamin D levels are associated with improved cognitive function. Include vitamin D-rich foods like fatty fish, fortified dairy products, and exposure to sunlight.

Magnesium

Magnesium plays a role in cognitive function and mood regulation. Incorporate magnesium-rich foods like nuts, seeds, leafy greens, and whole grains into your diet.

Caffeine Moderation

Some individuals with ADHD find caffeine exacerbates symptoms like restlessness and anxiety. Monitor your caffeine intake and consider reducing it if necessary.

Individualized Approach

Keep in mind that individual responses to diet can vary. What works for one person may not work for another. It's essential to pay attention to how specific foods affect your symptoms and adjust your diet accordingly.

Consult a Registered Dietitian

For personalized dietary guidance and meal planning, consider consulting a registered dietitian specializing in ADHD or neurodiverse diets. They can help create a tailored nutrition plan based on your specific needs.

Remember that dietary changes may not produce immediate results, and it's essential to approach them as part of a comprehensive ADHD management plan that may include behavioral therapy, medication (if prescribed), and other supportive strategies. Always consult with a healthcare professional or registered dietitian before making significant changes to your diet, especially if you have underlying medical conditions or specific dietary concerns.

Chapter 17

Meditation, Mindfulness and ADHD

Meditation and mindfulness practices have gained recognition as practical tools for managing the symptoms of ADHD. While these practices may not serve as standalone treatments, they can be valuable components of a comprehensive ADHD management plan.

Meditation is a mental practice that involves focused attention and heightened awareness to achieve a state of mental clarity, relaxation, and self-awareness. It often involves techniques like deep breathing, guided imagery, or mantra repetition.

Mindfulness is a specific form of meditation that emphasizes present-moment awareness without judgment. It involves paying attention to thoughts, feelings, sensations, and the surrounding environment with acceptance and without attempting to change or judge them.

Benefits of Meditation and Mindfulness for ADHD

Improved Focus and Attention

Meditation and mindfulness exercises can enhance the ability to sustain attention on a chosen focal point. This skill is precious for individuals with ADHD who often struggle with distractibility.

Emotion Regulation

Mindfulness promotes emotional regulation by helping individuals recognize and manage emotional reactions, reducing impulsive behaviors often associated with ADHD.

Reduced Stress and Anxiety

These practices are practical tools for reducing stress and anxiety, common co-occurring conditions in individuals with ADHD. Lower stress levels can improve overall well-being.

Enhanced Self-Awareness

Mindfulness encourages self-reflection and self-awareness, helping individuals better understand their thoughts, emotions, and behaviors. This self-awareness can lead to more effective self-management.

Better Impulse Control

Mindfulness practices encourage pausing and considering one's actions before reacting impulsively, promoting improved impulse control.

Improved Executive Functioning

Meditation and mindfulness can strengthen executive functioning skills, including organization, planning, and time management, which are often impaired in individuals with ADHD.

Enhanced Learning

By improving focus and attention, these practices can aid learning, making it easier for individuals with ADHD to absorb and retain information.

Practical Tips for Incorporating Meditation and Mindfulness

Start Small

Begin with short sessions, gradually increasing the duration as your ability to focus improves.

Consistency Matters

Regular practice is critical. Try to incorporate mindfulness exercises into your daily routine.

Guided Meditation

Utilize meditation apps, videos, or audio, which provide structured sessions and are accessible for beginners.

Mindful Breathing
Practice conscious breathing by focusing on your breath for a few minutes daily. This can be done anytime, anywhere.

Mindful Activities
Engage in everyday activities with mindfulness. Pay attention to your senses while eating, walking, or even doing household chores.

Mindfulness in School
If you have a child with ADHD, inquire whether their school offers mindfulness programs or consider introducing brief mindfulness exercises into their daily routine.

Seek Guidance
Consider working with a mindfulness teacher or therapist specializing in ADHD to receive personalized guidance and support.

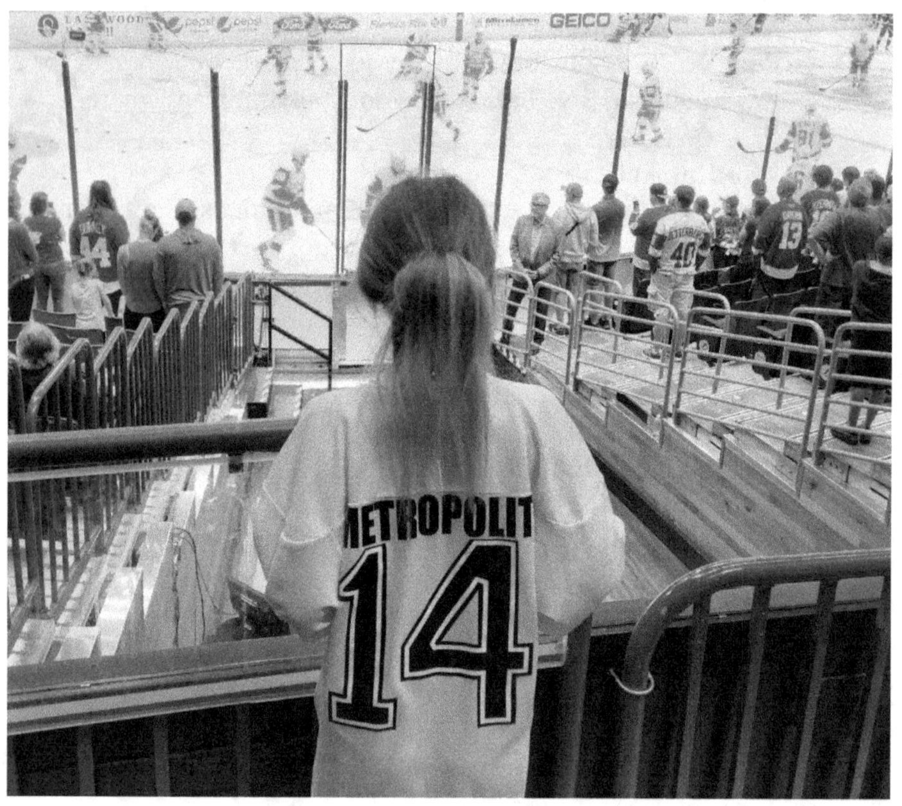

While meditation and mindfulness can be practical tools for managing ADHD symptoms, they may not replace other treatments for some individuals, such as behavioral therapy or medication. It's essential to consult with healthcare professionals and ADHD specialists to develop a comprehensive treatment plan tailored to individual needs.

I've tried meditation. My mom and I did it during the pandemic when I was homeschooled. I like it. Right now, I need help to fit it into my day. Routines should be flexible and adaptable. Here are two sample routines:

Morning Mindfulness Routine:
(Duration: Approximately 15-20 minutes)

Wake Up Mindfully (2 minutes)

Upon waking up, encourage them to take a moment to lie in bed, stretch, and become aware of their body and their surroundings.

Focus on taking a few deep, calming breaths to start the day with intention.

Mindful Breakfast (5 minutes)

While having breakfast, ask them to eat slowly and savor each bite. Encourage them to pay attention to their food's taste, texture, and smell. Discuss one thing they're looking forward to, or grateful for that day.

Guided Meditation (5 minutes)

Use a guided meditation app or video designed for children with ADHD. Focus on themes like grounding, calmness, and confidence. They can sit comfortably or lie down during the meditation, whichever feels more relaxing.

Mindful Breathing (3 minutes)

Practice deep breathing exercises. Count to four while inhaling, hold for four, and exhale for four. Repeat this pattern several times. Encourage them to notice how their body feels as they breathe deeply.

Set Intentions (2 minutes)

Before heading to school, ask them to set a positive intention for the day. This can be as simple as "I will stay focused in class" or "I will be kind to my classmates."

Evening Meditation and Relaxation Routine:
(Duration: Approximately 20-25 minutes)

Unwind After School (5 minutes)

When they return home from school, give them some time to decompress. This can include a snack and a brief chat about their day. Avoid overwhelming them with questions or tasks right away.

Mindful Art or Coloring (5 minutes)

Engage in a creative activity encouraging mindfulness, such as coloring or drawing. The focus should be on the process, not the result. Invite them to express their feelings through art if they're comfortable doing so.

Mindful Breathing and Body Scan (7 minutes)

Sit comfortably and guide them through a body scan meditation. This involves paying attention to each body part from head to toe, releasing tension, and promoting relaxation. Follow this with a few more minutes of mindful breathing.

Homework Break (2 minutes)

If they have homework, encourage them to take a short break. Stretch, drink water, or do a quick, mindful breathing exercise.

Bedtime Gratitude and Reflection (5 minutes)

Before bed, have them reflect on three things that went well during the day. Encourage them to express gratitude for these joyous moments. Discuss one thing they learned or experienced that day.

These routines provide structured opportunities for practicing meditation and mindfulness while accommodating the specific needs and challenges that may come with ADHD. Tailor the exercises as necessary to suit their preferences and schedule. The goal is to make mindfulness a vibrant and integrated part of their daily life.

Journaling

Keeping a journal can be valuable for kids with ADHD, even if they initially dislike it. It can help improve focus, organization, and self-expression. Here are some tips on how to make journaling a more enjoyable and practical experience for a child with ADHD who may not like it initially:

Make it Fun
Use a visually appealing journal or notebook with colors or designs that the child likes. Allow them to choose their journal materials, such as stickers, markers, or gel pens, to personalize their journal.

Set Realistic Expectations
Instead of insisting on daily journaling, establish a manageable schedule that fits their attention span and interests. It could be once a week or even less frequently if needed.

Use Prompts
Offer creative and engaging prompts to spark their interest. For example, ask about their favorite memories, dreams, or things they're excited about.

Focus on Positive Experiences
Please encourage them to write about positive experiences or achievements. Celebrating small victories can make journaling more rewarding.

Incorporate Visuals
Allow them to include drawings, doodles, or magazine clippings to make their journal visually appealing. Visual elements can be less intimidating than writing paragraphs.

Short and Sweet
Keep journal entries short. They might find long writing sessions overwhelming. A few sentences or bullet points can suffice.

Use Technology
Some children with ADHD may prefer digital journaling apps or voice recordings. These options provide a different medium for self-expression.

Focus on Interests
Tailor journaling topics to their interests. If they're passionate about a specific hobby or issue, encourage them to write about it.

Be Patient and Non-Judgmental
Avoid critiquing or correcting their journal entries. Make it clear that the journal is safe for them to express themselves without judgment.

Gradual Progress
Start with short journaling sessions and gradually increase the duration as they become more comfortable with the practice.

Celebrate Achievements
Acknowledge and celebrate milestones in their journaling journey. Positive reinforcement can motivate them to continue.

Share Your Journal
Consider sharing your journal entries to show them that journaling is a personal and beneficial practice for people of all ages.

Be Consistent and Patient
Encourage regularity, but be patient if they resist or skip journaling sessions. It's important to refrain from forcing the process.

Remember that journaling is a personal and adaptable practice. The key is to make it enjoyable, non-stressful, and a means of self-expression for the child. Over time, they may appreciate the benefits of journaling, even if they initially disliked the idea.

Chapter 18

Let's Talk About ADHD

I encourage everyone to talk more about ADHD to understand it better and help kids like me succeed. This condition is nothing to be ashamed of. This is not a fault or a punishment. ADHD means our brains don't work like a normal brain.

ADHD does not preclude success; many individuals with ADHD have achieved remarkable success in various fields. Here are a few famous people who have ADHD and have achieved great success:

Michael Phelps
The most decorated Olympian of all time has ADHD.
His hyperactivity as a child led his mother to introduce him to swimming as an outlet for his energy, which ultimately paved the way for his extraordinary swimming career.

Justin Timberlake
The multi-talented singer, actor, and entertainer Justin Timberlake has spoken openly about his ADHD diagnosis. He credits his hyper-focus ability, a common trait in people with ADHD, for his success in music and acting.

Sir Richard Branson
The billionaire entrepreneur and founder of the Virgin Group, Richard Branson, has ADHD. His ability to think outside the box and take risks has been instrumental in his business ventures.

Simone Biles
The renowned Olympic gymnast Simone Biles has ADHD. Her remarkable focus and dedication to her sport have led to numerous gold medals and record-breaking performances.

Will Smith

The actor, producer, and musician Will Smith has ADHD. He attributes his success to his ability to hyper-focus on tasks and his determination to excel.

Emma Watson

The actress best known as Hermione Granger in the Harry Potter films has discussed her ADHD diagnosis. Her intelligence and commitment to her craft have propelled her to success in the entertainment industry.

Adam Levine

The lead singer of Maroon 5, Adam Levine, has ADHD. He's known for his creativity and energetic stage presence.

Ty Pennington

The TV personality, carpenter, and designer Ty Pennington, known for shows like *Extreme Makeover: Home Edition*, has ADHD. His hyper-focus on his work has contributed to his success in the home improvement industry.

Solange Knowles

The singer, songwriter, and actress Solange Knowles has ADHD. She's celebrated for her creativity and unique artistic vision.

Jim Carrey

The actor and comedian Jim Carrey has ADHD. His boundless energy and comedic talent have made him a household name in the entertainment world.

These individuals demonstrate that ADHD can be a source of unique strengths and talents, contributing to their success in diverse fields. While ADHD may present challenges, it's not a barrier to achieving one's goals and significantly impacting the world.

Chapter 19

Finding a School

Looking for the best type of school for a child with inattentive type ADHD requires careful consideration and research. I'm in fifth grade, the end of elementary school. Next year, I go to middle school. Every adult in my family worries about middle school…especially my Gram. I have different feelings. I want to be around friends, but I also want to do well. Many of my friends will attend private or charter schools for middle school, or they will be homeschooled.

Let me say that just because a school is private and costs money doesn't mean it's better than a public school. You have to examine carefully what school choice is best for you.

Here are the pros and cons of three different types of schools—public schools, charter schools, and private schools—when considering them for inattentive ADHD students:

Public Schools Pros

Accessibility
Public schools are widely available and generally accessible to all students, including those with ADHD.

Legal Protections
Public schools are required by law to provide services and accommodations to students with disabilities under the Individuals with Disabilities Education Act (IDEA) and Section 504.

Diversity
Public schools often have diverse student populations, offering opportunities for students to interact with peers from various backgrounds.

Resource Support
Public schools may have access to special education services, Individualized Education Programs (IEPs), and other resources that can benefit students with ADHD.

Public School Cons:

Large Class Sizes
Many public schools have large class sizes, making it challenging for teachers to provide individualized attention to students with ADHD.

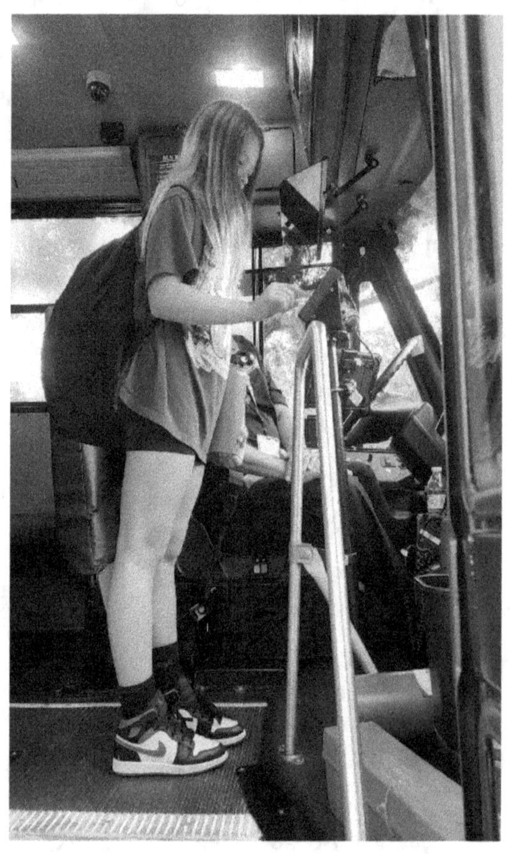

Limited Flexibility
Public schools may have less flexibility in tailoring instruction to meet the unique needs of students with ADHD.

Limited Choices
Students are generally assigned to public schools based on their residential address, limiting choices and options for parents seeking specific programs or approaches.

Bureaucracy
Public school systems can be bureaucratic, which may result in delays in evaluations and services.

Charter Schools Pros:

Variety of Approaches

Charter schools often offer specialized or alternative approaches to education, which can benefit students with ADHD who may thrive in non-traditional settings.

Smaller Class Sizes

Many charter schools prioritize smaller classes, allowing for more individualized attention.

Autonomy

Charter schools have greater freedom in curriculum development and teaching methods, enabling more flexibility to cater to the needs of students with ADHD.

Innovation

Charter schools may be more innovative in their educational approaches, including technology and individualized learning plans.

Charter School Cons:

Limited Availability

Charter schools are only available in some areas, and admission can be competitive, limiting access for some students.

Lack of Special Education Services

Some charter schools may have limited special education services or resources for students with ADHD.

Varying Quality

The quality of charter schools can vary widely, and not all charter schools may effectively meet the needs of students with ADHD.

Financial Constraints
Charter schools may have limited budgets and offer fewer extracurricular activities or resources than larger public schools.

Private Schools Pros:

Specialized Education
Private schools often offer technical programs for students with ADHD, including smaller class sizes and tailored teaching approaches.

Resources and Support
Some private schools have substantial resources and can provide comprehensive support, including tutoring and counseling.

Freedom of Choice
Parents can choose a private school that meets their child's needs and preferences.

Strong Parent Involvement
Private schools often encourage strong parental involvement, which can benefit students with ADHD.

Private School Cons:

Cost
Private schools can be expensive, and not all families can afford the tuition.

Limited Accessibility
Private schools may not be available in all areas, and admission can be selective.

Lack of Legal Protections
Private schools are not bound by the exact legal requirements for accommodating students with disabilities as public schools.

Varied Quality
The quality of private schools can vary widely, and not all private schools may effectively support students with ADHD.

Ultimately, the choice of school should be based on the individual needs and preferences of the student, as well as the available options in your area. It's essential to thoroughly research and visit schools, consider specific ADHD-related needs, and communicate openly with school administrators and teachers to make an informed decision. Additionally, seeking input from educational professionals and considering your family's financial situation is crucial in making the right choice.

Homeschooling and Virtual School
Other possibilities for a school choice option are homeschooling and virtual (online) school. Homeschooling or virtual school can be a viable options for a 6th-grade girl with ADHD, but it's essential to consider the potential advantages and disadvantages to determine a good fit. Let's start with homeschooling. Here are some pros and cons of homeschooling for a child with ADHD:

Homeschooling Pros:

Individualized Learning
Homeschooling allows for a highly individualized curriculum tailored to the child's specific learning style and pace, which can benefit ADHD students.

Flexible Schedule
Homeschooling offers flexibility in scheduling, allowing for breaks and adjustments based on the child's attention span and energy levels.

Reduced Distractions
The home environment can be less distracting than a traditional classroom, potentially enhancing focus and attention.

Personalized Accommodations
Parents can readily implement accommodations and strategies that work best for their child, such as frequent breaks, movement breaks, and specialized learning tools.

Reduced Anxiety
Homeschooling can reduce the social and performance-related anxiety some ADHD students experience in traditional school settings.

More One-on-One Attention
The student can receive more individualized attention from the parent or tutor, addressing specific learning challenges and providing immediate feedback.

Exploration of Interests
Homeschooling offers the flexibility to explore and delve deeply into students' interests and passions.

Homeschooling Cons:

Lack of Social Interaction
Homeschooling can lead to reduced social interaction with peers, potentially impacting the development of social skills and friendships.

Limited Extracurricular Activities
Homeschooled students may have fewer opportunities for extracurricular activities, sports, and clubs typically available in traditional schools.

Parental Time and Commitment

Homeschooling requires a significant time commitment from parents or caregivers, which may only be feasible for some families.

Potential for Isolation

Isolation from peers and a lack of exposure to diverse viewpoints may limit the child's social and cultural experiences.

Limited Access to Specialized Services

Homeschooled students may have limited access to special education services, speech therapy, or other resources typically available in public schools.

Parental Expertise

Parents may have expertise in some subjects, leading to potential gaps in the child's education or the need to hire tutors.

Legal Requirements

Homeschooling may be subject to specific legal requirements, including curriculum standards, standardized testing, and record-keeping, depending on the state or country.

Need for Discipline and Structure

Successful homeschooling often requires a structured daily routine and disciplined time management, which can be challenging for parents and students with ADHD.

Cost

Homeschooling can incur expenses for educational materials, resources, and potential tutoring or classes.

Transition Back to Traditional School

If the child eventually transitions back to traditional school, there may be an adjustment period and potential gaps in their academic preparation.

When considering homeschooling for a child with ADHD, it's crucial to weigh the pros and cons while also considering the child's specific needs, the resources available, and the family's ability to provide a supportive and structured learning environment. Additionally, consulting with education professionals and ADHD specialists can help make an informed decision that best serves the child's educational and developmental needs.

The biggest pro for homeschooling would be my Gram and Papa. My Papa is the only one who can teach me math, so I understand it. If my Gram and Papa took over homeschooling, I would benefit.

Virtual Schools

Virtual schools are also top-rated. In my state, there's a public virtual school option. Virtual schools for K-12 education have become increasingly popular in recent years, especially with advancements in technology and the global pandemic that accelerated the adoption of online learning. Like any educational model, virtual schools have their own set of pros and cons.

K-12 Virtual School Pros:

Flexibility
Virtual schools offer flexibility in terms of scheduling and location. Students can access their coursework from anywhere with an internet connection, allowing them to learn at their own pace and adapt their schedules to individual needs.

Personalized Learning
Virtual schools often use technology to provide customized learning experiences. Adaptive software and online assessments can tailor lessons to students' strengths and weaknesses, ensuring they get the support they need.

Access to a Wide Range of Courses
Virtual schools can offer a broader range of courses than traditional schools, including advanced placement (AP), dual

enrollment, and niche subjects that may not be available locally.

Safe Learning Environment
In the wake of the COVID-19 pandemic, virtual schools provided a safe alternative to in-person learning. This option can continue to be valuable during public health crises.

Reduced Commute
Virtual schools eliminate the need for long commutes, saving time and reducing stress for students and parents.

Individualized Pace
Students can progress through material at their own pace, allowing for mastery of concepts before moving on. This can be especially beneficial for students who need more time to grasp specific topics.

K-12 Virtual School Cons:

Lack of Social Interaction
Virtual schools can limit students' opportunities for face-to-face social interaction with peers and teachers, potentially impacting their social development.

Technological Barriers
Not all students can access technology and internet connectivity for virtual learning. This can exacerbate educational inequalities.

Self-Motivation Required
Virtual learning demands a high degree of self-discipline and motivation. Some students may need the structure and accountability provided by in-person classes.

Parental Involvement
Virtual education often requires parents to take on a more significant role in their child's learning, which can be challenging for working parents or those with limited educational backgrounds.

Isolation
Extended periods of virtual learning can lead to feelings of isolation and loneliness for some students, as they miss out on the social aspects of traditional schools.

Limited Extracurricular Activities
Many extracurricular activities, such as sports and clubs, are less accessible in virtual schools, potentially limiting students' opportunities for personal growth and skill development beyond academics.

Teacher-Student Relationship
Building and maintaining meaningful teacher-student relationships can be more challenging in virtual settings, which may impact the quality of instruction and support students receive.

Virtual schools for K-12 education offer significant advantages in terms of flexibility and personalized learning but also come with drawbacks related to social interaction, technological barriers, and the need for self-motivation. The effectiveness of virtual schooling depends on various factors, including the student's individual needs, the quality of the virtual school program, and the level of support available from parents and teachers.

Where to Start
To start the process of finding a school that fits your child's needs, start by clearly identifying your child's strengths and challenges related to ADHD. Make a list. Consider their learning style, any specific accommodations or strategies that have been helpful, as well as, their interests and preferences. Once you have this information

down, you're ready to start the search. Here are tips on how to proceed and what to look for:

Research School Options

Research different types of schools in your area, including public, private, charter, and specialized schools. Each type of school may offer additional resources and approaches to education.

Consult with Educational Professionals

Reach out to teachers, school counselors, or education specialists familiar with your child's needs. They can provide valuable insights and recommendations.

Visit Schools

Schedule visits to potential schools to observe the learning environment, meet with teachers and administrators and get a feel for the school culture. This includes virtual schools. Pay attention to class sizes, teaching methods, and available support services. This includes virtual schools. They provide virtual open-houses and additional ways to observe and get to know the staff and setting.

Consider Specialized Programs

Some schools offer specialized programs or schools-within-schools for students with ADHD or learning differences. Investigate whether these options are available in your area.

Review Academic Support Services

Inquire about the availability of academic support services, such as individualized education plans (IEPs) or 504 plans, which can provide accommodations tailored to your child's needs.

Evaluate Extracurricular Activities

Consider the availability of extracurricular activities that align with your child's interests. Engaging in extracurriculars can help improve focus and provide a sense of belonging.

Assess Class Size and Teacher Qualifications

Smaller class sizes and well-trained teachers who have experience working with students with ADHD can be advantageous. Ask about teacher-to-student ratios and teacher qualifications.

Discuss Discipline and Behavior Management

Inquire about the school's approach to discipline and behavior management. A supportive and understanding approach can benefit students with ADHD.

Consider Peer Relationships

Peer interactions are crucial for social development. Look for a school that fosters positive peer relationships and provides opportunities for socialization.

Seek Input from Your Child

Include your child in the decision-making process as much as possible. Their input on school preferences and concerns is valuable.

Review Testimonials and Reviews

Seek testimonials and reviews from parents of students with ADHD who have attended the schools you're considering. Their experiences can offer valuable insights.

Explore Transportation Options

Consider transportation logistics, especially if the school is not within walking distance. A long commute can add stress to a child's day.

Financial Considerations
Assess the financial implications of different school options, including tuition costs and available scholarships or financial aid.

Consult with Professionals
Consult educational psychologists or specialists who can provide assessments and recommendations to guide your decision.

Stay Involved and Advocate
Once your child is enrolled, stay actively involved in their education. Advocate for their needs and work collaboratively with teachers and administrators to ensure their success.

Chapter 20

Looking to the Future

As I grow up, I'm learning more about my ADHD and how to cope and even thrive with it. I'll talk about my dreams for the future and how I plan to make them come true, ADHD and all.

As a 5th-grade girl with inattentive ADHD, my future is filled with endless possibilities and exciting adventures. While there may be challenges, my unique strengths and the support of my family, friends, and educators will pave the path to a bright and promising future. Here's what I hope I can look forward to:

Academic Success
With the right strategies and support, I plan to do well enough in school to move to a post-secondary program. My creativity, out-of-the-box thinking, and ability to see the big picture will lead me to success. My passion for ice hockey and art will provide me with a career path.

Creative Ventures
My daydreams and imaginative mind will be my greatest assets. They'll lead me to explore the world of art and science. I want to create masterpieces that inspire and are helpful to others.

Lifelong Learning
I want to be a lifelong learner because I'm so curious. I don't think lifelong learning will take me to an academic career. I'm not one for the traditional classroom. However, I'll constantly seek new knowledge and explore new and exciting subjects.

Building Strong Friendships
My family and friends will continue to be my pillars of support. I'll forge meaningful relationships with those who appreciate my unique qualities and stand by me through thick

and thin. Together, we'll share countless adventures and unforgettable memories.

Overcoming Challenges

While challenges will arise, I'm resilient and determined to overcome them. As I grow, I'll develop essential life skills, such as time management and organization that will serve me well in adversity.

Personal Growth

As I journey through life, I want to discover more strengths and weaknesses. I'm very self-aware, enabling me to make informed choices and grow into a confident and capable young woman.

Making a Difference

My ability to think outside the box and my compassion for others will lead me to impact the world positively. I may champion causes close to my heart, advocate for those in need, or inspire others facing similar challenges.

Pursuing Passions

My unique perspective and talents will guide me to pursue my passions with vigor.

Loving and Being Loved

I hope, throughout my life, I'll experience love in its many forms. I'll cherish the love and support of my family and friends and may even get married and have my own children.

Embracing My ADHD Superpowers

I hope, as I grow older, I'll learn to harness my ADHD superpowers and turn them into strengths. My unique perspective, creativity, and ability to see the big picture may set me apart and make me a force to be reckoned with.

I must never forget that ADHD is just one facet of my incredible journey. My future is filled with remarkable experiences, personal growth, and the opportunity to leave my mark on the world. I want to embrace my ADHD, assert myself, and step boldly into the future, knowing that my potential is limitless.

One issue I will have that Gram is already thinking about is what diploma I will graduate with. In my state, if you don't get a specific score on the computerized state tests, you get an alternative certification. I imagine spending my last year of high school in another state that doesn't have such a ridiculous requirement so that I can get a standard diploma. Not all states are so uninformed about disabled kids. Many realize kids can be bright, but not do well on computerized state standardized tests. Some problems include:

Technical Issues
Computerized tests require students to have comfort and proficiency with technology. Technological difficulties such as computer glitches, slow internet connections, or unfamiliarity with the testing interface can impede performance.

Digital Divide
Not all students have equal access to technology and the internet at home. Disparities in access can lead to unequal preparation and test-taking experiences, affecting overall performance.

Keyboarding Skills
Younger students, in particular, may need more keyboarding skills, which can slow down their response times and make it challenging to complete the test within the allotted time.

Testing Anxiety
The transition from paper-and-pencil tests to computerized assessments can cause testing anxiety, as students may worry about accidentally clicking the wrong answer or navigating the interface. This anxiety can hinder their performance.

Lack of Familiarity

Some students may need to be more familiar with the computerized format of the test. They may need help navigating the questions, using features like highlighting or strikethrough or managing their time effectively.

Distractions

Computerized testing environments, especially in schools, may have distractions like noise from neighboring students, technical issues in the classroom, or discomfort with the computer setup.

Reading on Screens

Some students may need help reading lengthy passages or questions on a computer screen. They might be more accustomed to reading and annotating on paper.

Response Format

Computerized tests often require students to select answers using a mouse or keyboard, which can be less intuitive for some than simply filling in bubbles on a paper test.

Limited Practice

Students may need more exposure to computerized testing formats in their regular coursework or test preparation. Lack of practice can hinder their performance.

Adaptive Testing

Some computerized tests use adaptive algorithms that adjust the difficulty of questions based on a student's previous answers. If a student starts with challenging questions, it can demoralize and impact their overall performance.

Health and Well-Being
Physical discomfort, eye strain, or other health issues related to prolonged screen time can affect a student's ability to concentrate and perform well on computerized tests.

Teacher Training
The effectiveness of computerized testing can be influenced by the extent to which teachers are trained in facilitating and supporting students during these assessments.

Educators, administrators, and policymakers must recognize these challenges and appropriately support students. This support can include technology training, access to practice tests, creating comfortable testing environments, addressing technical issues promptly, and considering alternative testing methods for students who may struggle with computerized assessments. Ultimately, the goal should be to ensure that the testing mode does not unfairly disadvantage students and that their performance reflects their true abilities.

I'll never understand why adults are more concerned about winning elections than providing children with what they need.

Chapter 21

Above All Else, Stay Gritty

Grit is a term that describes a combination of determination, perseverance, resilience, and passion for long-term goals. It's a quality that plays a significant role in life and sports, and it can be precious for individuals, including ADHD girls, who face unique challenges and obstacles. Here's a closer look at what grit means in life and sports, especially for someone with ADHD:

Grit in Life:
Determination
Grit involves having a clear sense of what you want to achieve and deciding to work tirelessly toward those goals. For an ADHD girl, this may mean setting academic, personal, or social objectives and staying committed to them despite the potential for distraction or difficulty in staying on task.

Resilience
Grit helps individuals bounce back from setbacks and adversity. Living with ADHD often means dealing with focus, impulsivity, and organization challenges. Developing strength allows an ADHD girl to persevere when things get tough, learn from mistakes, and keep moving forward.

Passion
Grit is often fueled by passion and enthusiasm for a particular pursuit or life goal. When an ADHD girl discovers her interests and passions, it can motivate her to persist through challenges and setbacks.

Long-Term Perspective
Grit involves thinking beyond immediate gratification and focusing on long-term objectives. This might mean setting

goals that require sustained effort and breaking them down into smaller, manageable steps to maintain progress.

Grit in Sports:

Training and Improvement

In sports, grit means showing up for practice, even when motivation is low, and working consistently to improve skills and performance. ADHD girls can excel in sports by channeling their hyperactivity and energy into physical activities that they are passionate about.

Focus and Adaptation

Grit in sports includes maintaining focus during competition, adapting to changing game situations, and not becoming discouraged by mistakes. ADHD girls can use strategies like mindfulness and visualization to enhance their ability to stay focused.

Teamwork and Leadership

Grit in sports also involves being a supportive teammate, showing leadership, and contributing positively to the team's goals. Girls with ADHD can develop social skills and teamwork abilities beyond the playing field.

Overcoming Challenges

Sports often present various challenges, such as injuries or performance slumps. Grit helps athletes push through these obstacles, seek help when needed, and return stronger. ADHD girls can apply this same resilience to navigate their daily life challenges.

Goal Setting

Grit-driven athletes set clear and ambitious goals for themselves, whether winning a championship, improving personal records, or mastering a specific skill. Setting and pursuing these goals can be a powerful motivator.

For an ADHD girl, developing grit can be transformative. It allows her to harness her unique qualities and challenges, using them as sources of strength rather than limitations. With the proper support, guidance, and self-belief, she can apply grit to excel in life and sports, achieving her dreams and aspirations. Spirit is not about perfection but the determination to keep going, learn from setbacks, and grow stronger through the journey.

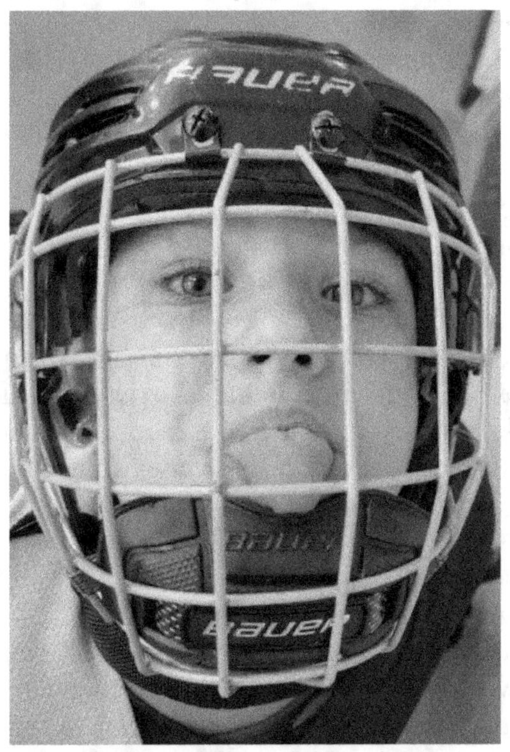

The Differences between Girls and Boys

There are presentation differences between boys with ADHD and girls with ADHD. Girls with ADHD may exhibit subtler signs of the disorder, such as forgetfulness, difficulty completing tasks, and trouble paying attention in class. They may often be perceived as quiet or shy, masking their restlessness and inner turmoil. Recognizing these subtleties is crucial for early intervention.

Social and Emotional Struggles
Girls with ADHD can face challenges in forming and maintaining friendships. They may struggle with impulse control, interrupting others in conversations, or grasping social nuances. Emotional dysregulation is common, leading to mood swings and outbursts and complicating social interactions.

Academic Performance
In the academic realm, girls with ADHD may display inconsistent performance. They might excel in subjects they are passionate about but need help with tasks that require sustained attention or organization. Their academic potential may be masked by inattention and homework completion difficulties.

Coexisting Conditions
Girls with ADHD often have comorbid conditions that may become apparent later in life. Anxiety and depression, for example, can develop due to the ongoing challenges they face. Recognizing and treating these coexisting conditions is vital for comprehensive care.

Masking and Camouflaging
Many girls with ADHD develop coping mechanisms to hide their difficulties. They may meticulously plan and organize their lives to compensate for their inattention, which can be exhausting. These strategies can delay diagnosis since the external appearance may not align with their internal struggles.

Delayed Diagnosis
Due to the atypical presentation and coping strategies of girls with ADHD, they may receive a diagnosis later than boys. Parents and educators may not suspect ADHD initially, attributing symptoms to personality traits rather than a medical condition.

Treatment and Support

Treatment should be individualized and holistic. Medication can effectively manage symptoms, but therapy, psychoeducation, and behavior interventions are equally important. Educators are crucial in supporting academic progress, while family support helps address day-to-day challenges.

Individualized Support

Recognizing each girl's unique strengths and challenges is essential. Some may excel in creative arts or sports; encouraging these interests can boost self-esteem and motivation. Tailoring interventions to their specific needs is more likely to yield positive results.

Education and Advocacy

Raising awareness about ADHD in girls among parents, educators, and healthcare professionals is a crucial advocacy point. This includes providing information on the gender-specific presentation of ADHD and promoting early identification to ensure timely intervention.

Emphasizing Strengths

Girls with ADHD often possess remarkable strengths such as creativity, resilience, and empathy. Encouraging and nurturing these talents can help build their self-esteem and self-confidence. By focusing on their positives, we can empower them to overcome challenges.

Understanding and supporting girls with ADHD requires a comprehensive approach, considering their unique experiences. It's crucial to look beyond stereotypes and assumptions, recognizing the individuality of each girl with ADHD and providing the tailored support they need to thrive in various aspects of their lives.

Aging with ADHD

Boys and girls with ADHD can continue to present differently as they grow up, but these differences can also become less pronounced or evolve. Several factors influence the way ADHD manifests in individuals as they age:

Hyperactivity, Inattention and Impulsivity
Hyperactivity tends to decrease with age in boys and girls, but other symptoms like inattention and impulsivity can persist into adulthood.

Hormonal Influences
Hormonal changes during adolescence and adulthood can affect the presentation of ADHD. For some girls, hormonal fluctuations may impact symptom severity, while boys may see changes related to their physical and emotional development.

Coping Mechanisms
As children with ADHD mature, they may develop coping strategies to manage their symptoms. Boys and girls may continue to employ different coping mechanisms, which can affect how their ADHD appears on the surface. For example, girls may become more skilled at masking their symptoms through increased organization and conscientiousness.

Socio-Cultural Factors
Societal and cultural expectations can influence how ADHD symptoms are perceived and expressed. Boys may be more likely to receive an early diagnosis due to the stereotypical presentation of hyperactivity. In contrast, girls may be overlooked or misdiagnosed due to their quieter, less disruptive symptoms.

Coexisting Conditions
The presence of coexisting conditions can also impact symptom presentation. For example, girls with ADHD may be more likely develop mood disorders like anxiety or depression,

which can overshadow or complicate recognizing ADHD symptoms.

Life Transitions
Major life transitions, such as entering college or starting a career, can affect how ADHD symptoms are experienced and managed. The demands of these transitions may exacerbate or mitigate certain aspects of the disorder.

Treatment and Intervention
Effective treatment and support can significantly influence how ADHD manifests in boys and girls as they grow up. Medication, therapy, and behavioral strategies can help individuals develop skills to manage their symptoms better.

It's important to note that while there can be gender-related differences in the presentation of ADHD, there is also a wide range of individual variation within each gender. Not all boys with ADHD will have the same symptoms or experiences, and the same holds for girls with ADHD. Early diagnosis, appropriate treatment, and ongoing support are essential for both genders to help individuals with ADHD thrive as they transition from childhood to adolescence and adulthood.

Self-Advocacy
We've touched on advocacy. Usually, parents are the first line of defense when advocating for their child's needs. As they age, though, kids with ADHD need to learn how to advocate for themselves. They must know exactly what they need to be successful in the world.

Self-advocacy is a crucial skill that empowers individuals to assert their needs, rights, and preferences. It's essential for people facing various challenges, including those with disabilities, chronic illnesses, or unique needs. Here are ten tips for advocating for oneself and some organizations that can provide additional support and guidance in self-advocacy:

Understanding Self-Advocacy

Self-advocacy involves actively voicing your concerns, desires, and requirements to meet your needs. It means taking responsibility for your well-being and actively participating in decisions that affect your life.

Know Your Rights

The first step in self-advocacy is knowing your rights. This includes understanding relevant laws, policies, and regulations that pertain to your situation. For instance, individuals with disabilities should be aware of the *Americans with Disabilities Act* (ADA) in the United States.

Educate Yourself

Gathering information about your condition or situation is essential. Be well-informed about your diagnosis, treatment options, and available resources. Knowledge is a powerful tool in advocating for yourself.

Clarify Your Goals:

Before advocating, define your objectives clearly. Please determine what you want to achieve, whether it's accessing specific accommodations, receiving better healthcare, or obtaining support services.

Effective Communication

Develop strong communication skills to express your needs and concerns clearly and assertively. Practice active listening and be open to collaborating with others.

Build a Support Network

Surround yourself with a supportive network of friends, family members, or mentors who can guide and encourage your advocacy efforts.

Self-Advocacy Training and Workshops

Numerous organizations offer self-advocacy training programs and workshops. These courses can teach practical skills, including communicating effectively with healthcare professionals or negotiating accommodations in educational or workplace settings.

Disability Rights Organizations

If you have a disability, consider contacting organizations like the *National Council on Independent Living* (NCIL) or the *Disability Rights Education & Defense Fund* (DREDF). These organizations offer resources, advocacy training, and legal support.

Patient Advocacy Groups

For individuals navigating the healthcare system, patient advocacy groups like the *Patient Advocate Foundation* or the *Alliance of Professional Health Advocates* can provide valuable guidance on accessing quality care and managing medical bills.

Mental Health Advocacy Organizations

Suppose you're dealing with mental health challenges. In that case, organizations like the *National Alliance on Mental Illness* (NAMI) offer advocacy resources, support groups, and educational materials to help you advocate for your mental health needs.

Education and Special Needs Advocacy

Parents and caregivers advocating for children with special needs in education can seek assistance from organizations such as the *Council of Parent Attorneys and Advocates* (COPAA) or the *Individuals with Disabilities Education Act* (IDEA) *Center*. These organizations can guide in securing appropriate educational services.

LGBTQ+ Advocacy Groups

LGBTQ+ individuals can turn to organizations like the *Human Rights Campaign* (HRC) for resources and support in advocating for equal rights and acceptance.

Legal Aid Services

Legal aid organizations can provide low-cost or pro bono legal assistance if your self-advocacy efforts involve legal issues. Look for local legal aid clinics or consult with national organizations like the *American Civil Liberties Union* (ACLU).

Online Communities and Forums

Engage with online communities and forums dedicated to your specific condition or situation. These platforms provide a space to share experiences, gather advice, and learn from others who have successfully advocated for themselves.

Persist and Be Patient

Self-advocacy can be lengthy, and you may encounter obstacles along the way. Persistence and patience are key. Keep pushing forward, seeking support when needed, and always appreciate the impact of your advocacy efforts.

Self-advocacy is a skill that can be developed and honed over time. Knowing your rights, being well-informed, communicating effectively, and seeking support from relevant organizations are essential to successful self-advocacy. Remember that advocating for yourself is an empowering act that can lead to positive changes in your life and the lives of others facing similar challenges.

Several organizations are dedicated to providing support, resources, and advocacy for children with ADHD and their families. Here are some prominent ones:

Children and Adults with Attention-Deficit/Hyperactivity Disorder (CHADD)

CHADD is one of the leading organizations focused on ADHD. They offer information, support groups, online forums, and resources for individuals with ADHD, parents, caregivers, and educators.

National Resource Center on ADHD (NRC)
NRC, a program of CHADD, provides comprehensive information and resources about ADHD. They offer fact sheets, webinars, and articles on various aspects of ADHD.

ADHD Awareness Month
ADHD Awareness Month is an annual campaign aimed at raising awareness about ADHD. They provide resources, events, and information to promote understanding and acceptance of ADHD.

ADDitude Magazine
ADDitude is a trusted source of information and support for individuals and families affected by ADHD. They offer articles, webinars, expert advice, and a community forum.

Understood.org
Understood.org provides resources and support for parents of children with learning and attention issues, including ADHD. They offer personalized tools and expert advice to help children succeed in school and life.

National Institute of Mental Health (NIMH)
NIMH provides information on ADHD research, treatment options, and clinical trials. Their website provides valuable resources for parents, educators, and healthcare professionals.

American Academy of Child and Adolescent Psychiatry (AACAP):
AACAP provides resources on ADHD, including fact sheets, practice guidelines, and information on finding a child and adolescent psychiatrist.

***National Center for Learning Disabilities* (NCLD)**
NCLD offers support for children with learning disabilities, including ADHD. They provide resources, advocacy tools, and information for parents and educators.

***National Alliance on Mental Illness* (NAMI)**
NAMI offers support and education for families with mental health conditions, including ADHD. They have local affiliates that provide support groups and educational programs.

Parent Training and Information Centers (PTIs)
These centers, funded by the U.S. Department of Education, provide information and support to parents of children with disabilities, including ADHD. Each state has its PTI, which can offer guidance on special education services and advocacy.

Your Local School District and Special Education Services
Many school districts have special education departments and resources to support children with ADHD. Parents can work with school staff to develop Individualized Education Programs (IEPs) or 504 plans tailored to their child's needs.

Local Support Groups
Look for local ADHD support groups in your area, often organized by community centers, hospitals, or nonprofit organizations. These groups provide opportunities for parents and children to connect with others facing similar challenges.

When seeking help and support for kids with ADHD, exploring multiple resources and organizations to find the most relevant and helpful information and services for your specific needs is essential. Additionally, consulting with healthcare professionals and educators can be instrumental in developing a comprehensive plan for managing ADHD in children.

ADHD and the Teenage Years

ADHD, or Attention Deficit Hyperactivity Disorder, is a neurodevelopmental condition that affects people of all ages, including teenagers. The teenage years are crucial in a person's life, marked by significant physical, emotional, and social changes. Adolescents with ADHD often face unique challenges during this phase of life. The teenage years, typically from ages 13 to 19, are characterized by rapid cognitive, emotional, and social development. These changes can interact with the symptoms of ADHD.

Challenges in School

Adolescents with ADHD may find it increasingly challenging to cope with the academic demands of middle and high school. They may need help with organization, time management, and staying focused on their studies.

Peer Relationships

Teenagers are forming their identities and navigating complex social dynamics. Adolescents with ADHD might encounter difficulties making and maintaining friendships, as impulsivity and inattention can affect their social interactions.

Emotional Regulation

Emotional regulation can be problematic for teenagers with ADHD. They may experience more intense mood swings, impulsivity in emotional responses, and difficulty managing frustration and anger.

Risk-Taking Behavior

Adolescents, in general, are more prone to engaging in risk-taking behaviors. However, teens with ADHD may be even more inclined towards impulsive decisions that can lead to negative consequences, such as substance abuse or reckless driving.

Medication Management

Adolescents with ADHD who take medication may face challenges independently adhering to their medication regimen. Parents and healthcare providers should work together to ensure proper medication management.

Transition to Independence

The teenage years are when adolescents seek more independence. Teens with ADHD may need additional support and guidance as they learn to manage responsibilities like chores and part-time jobs.

Driving Safety

For teenagers with ADHD, learning to drive can be a particularly critical issue. Impulsivity and inattention can increase the risk of accidents, making it essential for teens to receive specialized driver's education and ongoing support.

Coexisting Conditions

Adolescents with ADHD often have coexisting conditions, such as anxiety, depression, or learning disabilities. These conditions can complicate the management of ADHD and may require additional interventions.

Treatment Options

Treatment for ADHD in teenagers typically includes a combination of medication, behavioral therapy, and psychoeducation. Medication can help manage symptoms, while therapy provides coping strategies and skill-building.

Psychoeducation

Psychoeducation helps adolescents and their families understand ADHD better. It provides strategies for managing symptoms, improving communication, and fostering self-advocacy.

Parental Support

Parents of teenagers with ADHD play a critical role in providing emotional support, structure, and guidance. Setting clear expectations and maintaining consistent routines can help adolescents with ADHD thrive.

Educational Support

Schools can offer accommodations and support through Individualized Education Programs (IEPs) or 504 plans. These plans may include extended testing time, preferential seating, or modified assignments to help students with ADHD succeed academically.

Counseling and Therapy

Adolescents with ADHD may benefit from counseling or therapy to address emotional and social challenges. Cognitive-behavioral therapy (CBT) can help improve self-esteem and emotional regulation.

Self-Advocacy

Teaching teenagers with ADHD to advocate for themselves is crucial. This skill empowers them to effectively communicate their needs and preferences in academic and social contexts.

Peer Support Groups

Encouraging participation in peer support groups or therapy can help teenagers with ADHD connect with others facing similar challenges. These groups can reduce feelings of isolation and provide a sense of community.

Healthy Lifestyle Choices

Promoting healthy lifestyle choices, including regular exercise, a balanced diet, and sufficient sleep, can help manage ADHD symptoms in teenagers.

Future Planning
As teenagers approach adulthood, discussing plans, such as college or career choices, is essential. Adolescents with ADHD may need guidance in selecting pathways that align with their strengths and interests.

Hope and Resilience
While the teenage years can be challenging for adolescents with ADHD, many successfully navigate this phase of life with proper support, treatment, and resilience. With the right interventions and a supportive network, teenagers with ADHD can develop essential life skills and achieve their full potential.

The teenage years can be a period of growth and unique challenges for adolescents with ADHD. A multidisciplinary approach involving parents, educators, healthcare providers, and mental health professionals can help teenagers with ADHD overcome obstacles and build the skills needed to transition to adulthood successfully.

Chapter 22

Explore Your Options! You Can Succeed!

You are intelligent, talented, and capable. You must see the glass as half full and not half empty. I know I have problems that will be with me until the day I die, but I also have a lot going for me, and, as the saying goes, I want to be the best "me" I can be. I don't want to limit myself, and I don't want to assume that I can't do something and not even try.

Consider Your Options

ADHD girls, like all individuals, have a wide range of options for post-secondary education. Choosing an educational path that aligns with their interests, strengths, and goals is essential while considering their unique needs and challenges associated with ADHD. Here are several post-secondary education options that ADHD girls can explore:

Community College

Start at a two-year community college to complete general education requirements and explore academic interests before transferring to a four-year institution. Community colleges often offer smaller class sizes and more personalized attention, which can benefit students with ADHD.

Online or Hybrid Programs

Enroll in online or hybrid (combination of online and in-person) programs that offer flexibility and accommodate different learning styles. Digital tools and apps help with organization and time management in an online learning environment.

Trade or Technical Schools

Explore vocational or technical training programs in IT, culinary arts, or skilled trades. These programs often have hands-on learning opportunities, which can be engaging for students with ADHD.

Art, Music, or Creative Schools

Attend specialized institutions for those passionate about the arts, music, or creative fields. Such schools often emphasize creativity and can be a good fit for students with artistic talents.

Gap Year Programs

Take a gap year to explore interests, work, volunteer, or gain life experience before committing to formal post-secondary education. Gap years can provide valuable clarity about career goals and interests.

Non-Traditional Paths

Explore alternative educational paths, such as apprenticeships, internships, or certificate programs, which can lead to fulfilling careers without a traditional degree.

Supportive Programs and Colleges

Explore colleges and universities with specialized support programs for students with ADHD or learning disabilities. These programs often provide tutoring, counseling, and academic coaching tailored to individual needs.

Adult Education and Continuing Education

Take adult education courses or enroll in continuing education programs to acquire new skills, change careers, or pursue personal interests.

Self-Paced Learning and Personal Development

Embrace self-directed learning through online courses, workshops, or self-help resources. Focus on personal development and acquiring skills relevant to career goals.

It's crucial for ADHD girls to carefully research and consider their options, visit campuses or attend information sessions, and seek guidance from mentors, counselors, and support networks. Additionally, understanding their rights to accommodations under the *Americans with Disabilities Act* (ADA) and *Section 504* of the *Rehabilitation Act* can help them receive the support they need to succeed in their chosen educational path. Ultimately, the right choice will depend on individual interests, strengths, and aspirations, and it may involve a combination of different educational experiences over time.

Fighting the "I am dumb" Syndrome

I've already talked about the fact that I've been tested, and I'm not dumb. My problem is that, in school, I can feel pretty dumb, especially in math. I am the slowest to come up with answers; I get my work wrong and must be retaught.

Fighting the "I am dumb" syndrome or negative self-perception at school can be challenging, but it's crucial to building confidence and achieving academic success. Here are some strategies to help combat these feelings:

Recognize Negative Self-Talk

The first step is to become aware of when you're engaging in negative self-talk. Pay attention to the thoughts and beliefs reinforcing the "I am dumb" syndrome.

Challenge Negative Thoughts

Whenever you catch yourself thinking negatively about your abilities, challenge those thoughts. Ask yourself if there's evidence to support them or if they are based on assumptions.

Practice Self-Compassion

Treat yourself with the same kindness and understanding you would offer to a friend facing similar challenges. Remember that everyone makes mistakes and has areas where they struggle.

Set Realistic Expectations

Set achievable goals and expectations for yourself. Don't compare your abilities to others; everyone has strengths and weaknesses.

Seek Support

Talk to a trusted teacher, counselor, or a supportive adult about your feelings. They can provide guidance, reassurance, and resources to help you overcome self-doubt.

Focus on Effort, Not Perfection

Shift your focus from being perfect to putting in your best effort. Mistakes are opportunities for growth and learning.

Develop Study Strategies

Work on developing effective study strategies that suit your learning style. This can help improve your understanding of the material and boost your confidence.

Use Positive Affirmations

Create and repeat positive affirmations that counteract negative self-perceptions. For example, "I am capable of learning and improving" or "I am a smart and determined student."

Build on Strengths

Identify your strengths and interests, and use them as a foundation for boosting your confidence. Success in one area can positively impact your overall self-esteem.

Stay Organized

Organize your schoolwork, assignments, and deadlines. Being organized can help reduce feeling overwhelmed and boost your sense of control.

Seek Learning Support
If you're struggling academically, feel free to seek help from teachers, tutors, or academic support services. These resources are there to assist you in understanding and mastering the material.

Practice Growth Mindset
Embrace a growth mindset, believing your abilities can improve through effort and learning. Understand that intelligence is not fixed.

Celebrate Small Wins
Acknowledge and celebrate your achievements, no matter how small they may seem. This positive reinforcement can boost your self-esteem over time.

Stay Persistent
Persistence is vital to overcoming challenges. Keep trying, even when things get tough, and remember that setbacks are part of the learning process.

Combating negative self-perceptions takes time and effort. Be patient with yourself and seek support when needed. With dedication and the right mindset, you can overcome the "I am dumb" syndrome and develop greater confidence in your academic abilities.

Chapter 23

Negative Outcomes Aren't Inevitable

I've been as positive as I can be about my ADHD and my academic struggles, but it's hard. Sometimes, my family is the only reason I can put a smile on my face and move on.

While ADHD is a treatable condition, it's associated with various challenges that can lead to negative statistics and outcomes in certain areas of life. It's important to note that not every individual with ADHD experiences these difficulties to the same extent, and many people with ADHD lead successful and fulfilling lives. However, here are some statistics and potential adverse outcomes associated with ADHD to be aware of:

Academic Underachievement
According to some studies, individuals with ADHD are at a higher risk of academic difficulties, including lower grades, lower standardized test scores, and dropping out.

Employment Challenges
Adults with ADHD may face challenges in the workplace, including difficulties with time management, organization, and maintaining consistent focus. Some studies suggest higher rates of unemployment and underemployment among individuals with ADHD.

Risk-Taking Behavior
Those with ADHD may be more prone to risky behaviors, such as substance abuse or reckless driving, which can lead to negative consequences. Research has shown a correlation between ADHD and an increased risk of substance abuse and addiction, including alcohol, tobacco, and illicit drugs.

Impulsivity, risk-taking behavior, and self-medication may contribute to these issues.

Coexisting Conditions
ADHD often coexists with other mental health conditions like anxiety and depression. These comorbidities can complicate treatment and increase the overall burden on individuals.

Relationship Struggles
ADHD symptoms, particularly impulsivity and inattention, can strain personal relationships. Individuals with ADHD may struggle with communication, forgetfulness, and emotional regulation, impacting family and social dynamics.

Legal Issues
Some individuals with untreated or unmanaged ADHD may encounter legal issues related to impulsive behavior, such as traffic violations or legal disputes.

Health and Lifestyle Challenges
Poor impulse control and difficulties with self-regulation can contribute to unhealthy lifestyle choices, including poor diet, lack of exercise, and inconsistent sleep patterns, which may lead to health issues.

Financial Problems
Managing finances can be challenging for individuals with ADHD due to difficulties with budgeting, impulse buying, and maintaining financial records.

Emotional and Self-Esteem Issues
Repeated experiences of underachievement, criticism, or perceived failure can impact self-esteem and lead to feelings of frustration and low self-worth.

Increased Risk of Suicide
Research has suggested a higher risk of suicidal ideation and suicide attempts among individuals with ADHD, particularly during adolescence and early adulthood. This may be linked to the emotional and psychological struggles that some individuals with ADHD face, such as depression, anxiety, and feelings of frustration or isolation.

It's important to emphasize that these statistics and outcomes are not predetermined or inevitable for individuals with ADHD. With early diagnosis, appropriate treatment, and support, many individuals with ADHD can mitigate these challenges and lead successful lives. Effective treatments for ADHD often include a combination of behavioral therapies, medication, and educational support.

Furthermore, some individuals with ADHD possess unique strengths, such as creativity, innovation, and the ability to think outside-the-box. By harnessing these strengths and addressing challenges, individuals with ADHD can achieve positive outcomes and contribute to various life aspects.

While it's essential to recognize these challenges, it's equally important to stress that adverse outcomes are not inevitable, and many individuals with ADHD can lead fulfilling lives with the proper support and interventions.

Chapter 24

Understanding Hope

Hope is a complex psychological construct encompassing beliefs in one's ability to set and achieve goals, overcome adversity, and maintain a positive outlook on the future. It consists of two main components agency and pathways.

Agency refers to the belief in one's capacity to initiate actions, make choices, and exert control over their life circumstances. For individuals with ADHD, agency translates into their ability to manage symptoms, seek help, and make positive changes.

Pathways involve the identification of potential routes and strategies to reach one's goals. It is about finding solutions, alternatives, and support systems that can lead to success. For individuals with ADHD, pathways can include seeking treatment, building effective routines, and tapping into their unique strengths.

The Impact of Hope on ADHD Individuals

Academic Achievement and Motivation

Hope is a potent motivator in academic settings. Children with ADHD who possess hope are more likely to set and pursue educational goals, engage in effective study strategies, and persist in facing challenges. They are driven by the belief that their efforts will lead to success.

Improved Mental Health and Well-being

Hope contributes to improved mental health outcomes for individuals with ADHD. It acts as a buffer against depression, anxiety, and feelings of helplessness. Hopeful individuals are better equipped to cope with stress and adversity.

Resilience and Coping Strategies

Hope nurtures resilience, the ability to bounce back from setbacks. ADHD individuals with hope are more likely to develop effective coping strategies, adapt to changing circumstances, and maintain a positive outlook despite difficulties.

Enhanced Self-Esteem and Self-Perception
Hope fosters positive self-esteem and self-perception. Children and adults with ADHD who believe in their abilities and see a hopeful future are more likely to view themselves positively, embracing their strengths and talents.

Positive Effects on Relationships
Hope extends to interpersonal relationships. Individuals with ADHD who maintain hope are better equipped to build and sustain positive relationships with family, friends, and colleagues. Their optimism and determination can inspire and motivate those around them.

Fostering and Cultivating Hope
Education and Awareness: Raising awareness about ADHD and educating individuals about the condition can help dispel misconceptions and create a foundation of understanding, which is crucial for fostering hope.

Effective Treatment
Access to appropriate treatment, including behavioral therapies and medication when necessary, can significantly improve symptom management and enhance hope for better outcomes.

Support Systems
Building supportive networks of family, friends, and professionals who understand and encourage individuals with ADHD can be a powerful source of hope.

Goal Setting and Achievement

Helping ADHD individuals set realistic goals, both short-term and long-term, and celebrating their achievements along the way reinforces hope and motivation.

Embracing Individual Strengths

Recognizing and celebrating the unique strengths and talents of individuals with ADHD empowers them to see themselves as capable.

Promoting a Growth Mindset

Encouraging a growth mindset, where challenges are seen as opportunities for growth and learning, fosters resilience and hope.

Hope is not just a fleeting emotion but a vital resource that can transform the lives of children and adults with ADHD. By believing in their ability to set and achieve goals, overcome challenges, and shape a positive future, individuals with ADHD can navigate life's complexities with optimism and resilience. Understanding the importance of hope and actively fostering it within the ADHD community is fundamental to improving well-being and success for all.

Hope for People Who Love You

ADHD doesn't just impact the one suffering. It touches everyone that loves that person. We love our children and grandchildren and want them to have a smooth, happy, and healthy life unhindered by disease or misfortune. Unfortunately, that isn't always possible.

Parenting a child with ADHD can be challenging, but it's also an opportunity to provide essential support and nurture hope. Hope is a powerful asset for children with ADHD, helping them navigate the complexities of the condition, build resilience, and envision a bright future. Parents and families play a crucial role in keeping hope alive for the child with ADHD, emphasizing the importance of understanding, patience, and active support.

Understanding ADHD as a Family

Education and Awareness
To foster hope effectively, families must first understand what ADHD is and how it manifests. This knowledge helps parents and caregivers recognize and empathize with their child's challenges.

Dispelling Myths and Reducing Stigma
Families can help dispel common myths and misconceptions about ADHD within the family unit and the wider community. By addressing stigma, they create a more supportive environment for their child.

Providing Emotional Support

Open and Non-Judgmental Communication
Families should create a safe space for open communication where the child can express their feelings, fears, and frustrations without fear of judgment. Active listening is critical.

Positive Reinforcement
Acknowledging and celebrating even small achievements can boost a child's self-esteem and instill hope. This positive reinforcement motivates them to keep trying.

Promoting a Growth Mindset
Encouraging a growth mindset, where challenges are seen as opportunities for growth and learning, helps the child develop resilience and maintain hope in the face of setbacks.

Navigating Treatment and Support

Accessing Professional Help

Families play a vital role in seeking professional evaluation and treatment for their child's ADHD. Access to therapies, such as behavioral interventions and, in some cases, medication, can significantly improve symptom management and hope for a better future.

Consistency in Treatment Plans

Consistency in following treatment plans, including medication schedules and therapy sessions, is crucial. Families should work together to ensure the child receives the support they need.

Individualized Support

Recognizing that each child with ADHD is unique, families should tailor support to their child's needs, strengths, and challenges.

Building Structure and Routine

Establishing Daily Routines

Creating structured daily routines helps children with ADHD manage their time effectively and reduces feelings of chaos and overwhelm.

Setting Clear Expectations

Families should set clear, age-appropriate expectations and communicate them to the child. Clear expectations help reduce frustration and foster a sense of control.

Promoting Independence and Self-Advocacy

Teaching Self-Management Skills

Families can gradually teach their children essential self-management skills, such as organization, time management, and impulse control. These skills empower the child and boost self-confidence.

Encouraging Self-Advocacy
Families should encourage their children to express their needs, advocate for accommodations when necessary, and communicate with teachers and peers about their ADHD. This fosters a sense of agency and hope.

Parents and families play a central role in nurturing hope for children with ADHD. By understanding the condition, providing emotional support, facilitating treatment access, creating structure, and promoting independence, families can empower their children to navigate the challenges of ADHD with resilience and optimism. Keeping hope alive is not only beneficial for the child's well-being, but also contributes to their overall success and fulfillment in life.

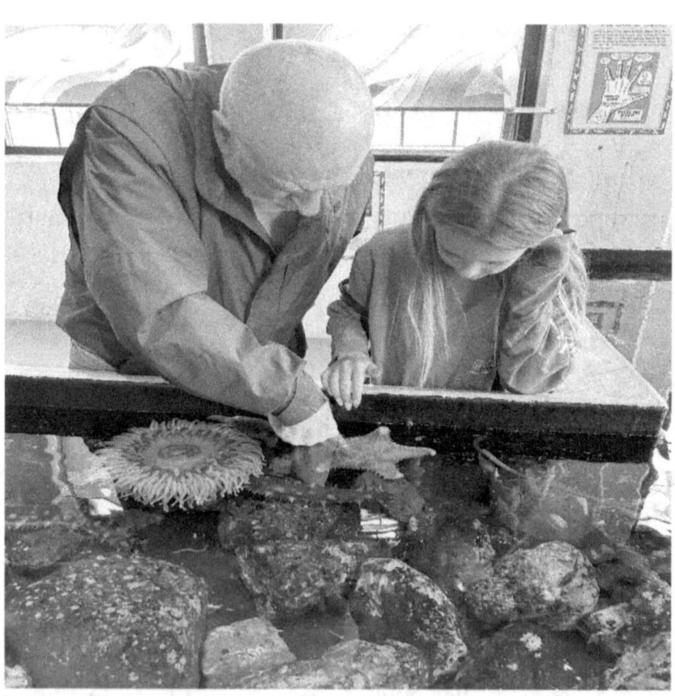

Taking Care of Yourself as a Parent

Parenting a child with ADHD can be challenging, but parents must maintain a positive outlook, a sense of hope and take care of themselves. Here are some strategies to help parents stay positive, resilient and healthy on their parenting journey:

Educate Yourself

Knowledge is power. Learn as much as possible about ADHD, its symptoms, treatment options, and strategies for managing it. Understanding the condition can help demystify it and reduce feelings of frustration or helplessness.

Connect with Support Groups

Joining support groups for parents of children with ADHD can be incredibly helpful. Sharing experiences, tips, and challenges with others who can relate can provide a sense of community and understanding.

Practice Self-Care

Caring for a child with ADHD can be emotionally and physically draining. Make self-care a priority. Take breaks, seek support from friends and family, and engage in activities that rejuvenate you.

Embrace Flexibility

Understand that flexibility is critical when parenting a child with ADHD. Plans may change, and challenges may arise. Adaptability and patience are essential.

Stay Calm and Consistent

Consistency in routines and expectations is crucial. Stay calm when addressing challenging behaviors, and model the behavior you want to see in your child.

Practice Mindfulness
Mindfulness techniques, such as deep breathing or meditation, can help you manage stress and stay present in the moment, reducing feelings of overwhelm.

Focus on Progress, Not Perfection
Understand that progress may be gradual. Celebrate the journey and the improvements your child makes rather than aiming for perfection.

Communicate Openly
Maintain open and honest communication with your child. Please encourage them to express their thoughts and feelings and listen without judgment.

Be Kind to Yourself
Parenting a child with ADHD can be challenging, and no one is perfect. Forgive yourself for your mistakes, and remember you are doing your best.

Take One Day at a Time
Don't overwhelm yourself by thinking too far ahead. Take each day as it comes, and focus on what you can do today to support your child.

Seek Professional Support for Yourself
Don't hesitate to seek therapy or counseling if you find that managing your child's ADHD is taking a toll on your mental health. A therapist can provide coping strategies and emotional support.

Remember that you are not alone in this journey; resources and communities are available to support you. With patience, understanding, and a positive outlook, you can provide the love and guidance your child with ADHD needs to thrive.

It's also essential for parents not to cast self-blame for having a child with ADHD. ADHD is a neurodevelopmental condition that results from a complex interplay of genetic, environmental, and neurological factors. It is not the result of parenting or any actions on the part of the parents. Here are some reasons why self-blame is unwarranted and counterproductive:

Biological Nature of ADHD
ADHD is primarily a genetic and neurological condition. Parenting styles, lack of discipline, or any perceived shortcomings of the parents do not cause it.

No Control over Genetic Factors
Parents do not have control over the genetic factors that contribute to ADHD. It is not something that can be prevented or caused by parental actions.

ADHD is Common
ADHD is a relatively common condition affecting millions of children worldwide. It is not a reflection of parenting skills or parental "fault."

Diverse Range of ADHD Experiences
Children with ADHD have many experiences and challenges. Blaming oneself does not consider the inherent variability in how ADHD manifests.

Focus on Support and Understanding
Instead of self-blame, parents can focus on providing their children with the support, understanding, and resources they need to thrive. Effective management of ADHD involves learning about the condition, seeking appropriate treatments, and fostering a supportive and loving environment.

Parents should avoid self-blame and instead channel their energy and efforts into understanding, accepting, and supporting their child with ADHD. A compassionate and proactive approach and access to appropriate resources can significantly impact the child's life and the family's overall well-being.

Chapter 25

A Parable

Once upon a time, in a small village lived a girl named MG. She was a bright and creative soul, always lost in her world of imagination. However, MG had a unique challenge – she had inattentive ADHD. While she was full of brilliant ideas, her thoughts often danced around like fireflies, making it challenging to focus on any one thing for long.

MG's classmates excelled in school as she grew older, earning praise and admiration from teachers and parents. Meanwhile, MG's forgetfulness and difficulty paying attention left her feeling different and inadequate. Her report cards were a patchwork of highs and lows, reflecting her inconsistent academic performance.

One sunny afternoon, as MG wandered by a tranquil pond, she met an older man named Mr. Alden, known for his wisdom. She shared her struggles and frustrations with him, tears glistening.

Mr. Alden smiled gently and said, "MG, your ADHD may make you different, but it doesn't define your worth or potential. It can be your greatest gift. Your mind is like a garden with a thousand flowers, each blooming in its own time. Embrace your uniqueness, and you will find your path to success."

MG took Mr. Alden's words to heart. Instead of trying to fit into the mold created by others, she decided to create her own. She realized her creativity thrived when she allowed her mind to wander freely. She began to carry a notebook with her, jotting down every idea that fluttered through her thoughts.

MG discovered her ability to think outside the box was valuable in time. She started working on projects that required innovation and creativity and excelled. Her inconsistency became an advantage as she was not bound by conventional thinking. She could adapt to different tasks and solve problems from unique angles.

With perseverance, she turned her creativity into a successful career. She became an inventor known for her groundbreaking ideas. Her inventions helped people in ways they had never imagined. MG's name spread far and wide, and she was celebrated not for fitting in but for standing out.

People marveled at how MG's inattentive ADHD had become the source of her success. She proved that being different could be an extraordinary strength. She also became an advocate through her journey, helping others with ADHD recognize their potential and embrace their uniqueness.

MG's parable teaches us that success isn't determined by how well one fits into a predefined mold. Instead, it's about embracing our individuality and using our unique qualities to carve our paths in life. Like MG, we can turn our perceived weaknesses into our greatest strengths and inspire others to do the same.

As MG's grew, she always remembered the wisdom Mr. Alden had shared with her by the pond. She knew that success wasn't just about achieving personal goals and giving back to her community.

MG established a foundation that supported children with learning differences, including ADHD. She wanted to ensure that every child had the chance to embrace their unique abilities, just as she had. Her foundation provided resources, educational programs, and scholarships to empower young minds to reach their full potential.

One day, a young boy named Ethan, who also had ADHD, came across MG's foundation. He had always struggled in school and felt like an outcast. Encouraged by his parents, he attended one of the foundation's programs.

Under the guidance of caring educators who understood his challenges, Ethan thrived. The program encouraged his creativity and helped him develop strategies to manage his ADHD effectively. He started believing in himself and his abilities.

Years passed, and Ethan grew up to be a brilliant scientist. His groundbreaking discoveries in neuroscience helped unlock the mysteries of the human brain and led to innovative treatments for various learning differences, including ADHD. He credited his success to the support and inspiration from MG's foundation.

MG and Ethan's stories symbolized hope and resilience for countless children and families facing similar challenges. They demonstrated that with determination, self-acceptance, and the support of a caring community, anyone could turn adversity into an opportunity for success.

The legacy of MG and Ethan continued to shine as a beacon of light, guiding generations of young minds to embrace their uniqueness, pursue their dreams, and positively impact the world. The small village, once unaware of the power of differences, became a place that celebrated the diversity of talents and abilities within its community, thanks to the enduring influence of one girl with inattentive ADHD and one young scientist who refused to be defined by their challenges.

Chapter 26

I Am Gram

I am Gram, and this chapter is all mine. I wanted to end this little book with my thoughts and concerns. Although I have peppered my observations and ideas throughout this collaboration between my granddaughter and myself, I wanted to highlight the things that keep me up at night.

ADHD is brutal. It robs those who have it of the ability to function as normally as those who don't have it. It plays havoc with executive functioning, making those afflicted look less than capable. It can demoralize to the point of hopelessness.

My granddaughter is in 5th grade; she is only ten years old. In her mind, she is one of the dumb kids in class. We talk about the fact that her brain works differently and that she's smart and talented. However, when she has to, again, go to the back of the room to receive special help, her disabilities are reinforced. She's different, and it can be a difference that hurts.

I spent my life as an educator. I was an educational consultant for a state agency and worked with students with special needs. I evaluated them for special education and placed them in special programs if they qualified. I worked with and consulted with teachers and administrators. I sat on the other side of the table.

I now get to experience being the non-educator, the grandparent, the person who may be perceived by school personnel as not knowledgeable. I'm now the advocate, the person who lives with the daily struggles of a child saddled with the burden of ADHD.

I've encountered every kind of educator. The ones who see me as an equal and who have the skill set to provide pertinent information about ADHD in general and my granddaughter in particular.

We talk about the different types of education in our book. Is public better? Private? Charter? Virtual? I have scoured the internet reading about each type of school and what might be best for my granddaughter. How do you find the perfect marriage of highly skilled and caring? Does that exist?

Beyond the educator's skill set, has to be the heart of a person who loves kids and is passionate about teaching. The two go hand-in-hand.

They must understand this disability; they must be current, and they must be masters. Can this be found at this pay-scale?

I have found that school districts do a spectacular job of formulating mission statements touting their beliefs that all children are precious and deserve the best. Here are a couple of real-life mission statements:

"To provide an education and supports that enable each student to excel as a successful and responsible citizen."

"The mission of the state education system is to increase the proficiency of all students within one seamless, efficient system, by allowing them the opportunity to expand their knowledge and skills through learning opportunities and research valued by students, parents, and communities."

Don't these mission statements sound grand? Sign me up. Unfortunately, the mission statements don't always align themselves with reality. Teachers are very poorly paid in my state. Teacher turnover is great. Teachers don't appear to be respected or appreciated by those who employ them.

I have followed up on concerns to the state level and have been ignored. From my experience, the mission statements of those offices I have dealt with might very well be:

"We have too much to do to individualize instruction for your child. Reaching full potential is for the child who presents us with no problems."

Teachers need to be better trained, better supported, and better paid. We are the living embodiment of "you get what you pay for." This isn't an environment where the best choose to be employed or stay employed. We have a crisis in education that well-crafted mission statements cannot cover up, and parents and children suffer.

The internet is full of attorneys offering their services to parents of disabled children. This is a lucrative area. So, what does a family do with a child with special needs? Who has the training and support system to provide that child with an education that will help them reach their full potential? The simple answer is, "I don't know."

Some companies specialize in finding the right school for your child. Most parents cannot afford them. Some companies specialize in providing individualized instruction. Most parents cannot afford them.

The need is great, but the ability to access these services is very difficult for most families. Sitting on the other side of the table, I have learned many things:

- I know more about my granddaughter than any of her teachers.
- I have more expertise in the curriculum than any of her teachers.
- I have more expertise in individualizing instruction than any of her teachers.
- I have a much better understanding of special education law than anyone at the school.
- I'm not considered a partner who can provide important information; I'm considered a nuisance and a threat to the status quo.

I was an education consultant for decades. I spent a lot of time working with parents. I found that they could provide important information. If parents were angry, it was because they were afraid. Fear drives anger. Fear that your child will not succeed at anything. We have to partner with the families of disabled children or we'll continue to provide substandard services, and children will continue to fail by the scores.

This chapter is not a dissertation on test scores, but parents need to inform themselves about their district and state trends on state and federal. The pandemic played a part in the declines, but alarms were sounding before the pandemic began. As far as I can see, the dismal performance on these tests simply provided bureaucrats with another platform to spout mission statements and platitudes.

My granddaughter's family is committed to providing her with every opportunity to help her be successful. We have our own mission statement:

"We will work to provide a learning environment in which our granddaughter can excel academically, socially, and emotionally. We will provide her with fertile ground to become the best person she can be and meet the demands of the 21st-century adult."

Being a parent or grandparent of a child, especially a girl, with ADHD can be a complex and emotional experience. It often involves a mix of challenges, frustrations, joys, and moments of pride. Here are some common feelings and experiences you might have:

Concern: You may worry about your child or grandchild's well-being, their academic performance, and their social interactions. ADHD can make these aspects of life more challenging, and it's natural to be concerned about their future.

Frustration: You might feel frustrated when it seems like your child or grandchild is struggling with tasks or behaviors that come more easily to others. The impulsivity and inattention associated with ADHD can sometimes lead to challenging behaviors and difficulties with tasks like homework.

Empathy: You may have a deep understanding of your child's struggles and empathize with their daily challenges. This can create a strong bond as you work together to find solutions and support them in managing their ADHD.

Pride: Witnessing your child or grandchild's accomplishments, no matter how small they may seem to others, can fill you with immense pride. Their successes, even in the face of adversity, can be incredibly rewarding.

Advocacy: You may find yourself advocating for your child or grandchild in various settings, such as schools, doctors' offices, or with family and friends. Advocacy can be both empowering and exhausting, but it's essential to ensure they receive the support they need.

Learning: Being a parent or grandparent of an ADHD child can be an ongoing learning experience. You may need to educate yourself about ADHD, treatment options, and effective strategies for managing symptoms. This learning journey can be both challenging and enriching.

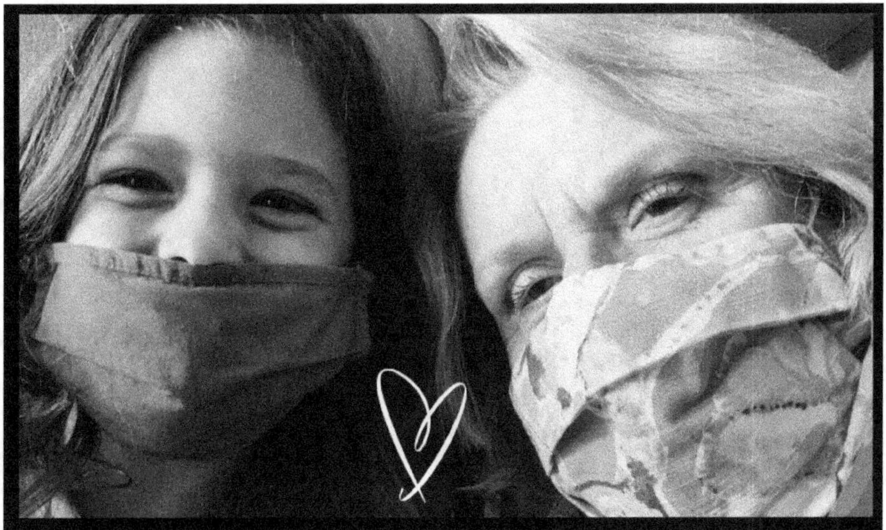

Patience: ADHD can bring about impulsive behaviors and difficulties with focus, which can test your patience. It's essential to cultivate patience as you work with your child or grandchild to help them develop coping mechanisms.

Love and Support: Regardless of the challenges, your love and support are crucial to your child's well-being. Your unwavering belief in their abilities can be a source of strength for them.

Hope: It's important to maintain hope for your child's future. With the right support, interventions, and coping strategies, many children with ADHD go on to lead successful, fulfilling lives.

Connection: You may feel a unique connection with your child or grandchild due to the shared experiences and challenges associated with ADHD. This bond can be a source of comfort and understanding.

Being the parent or grandparent of an ADHD child means navigating a journey with its ups and downs. You are her champion, her advocate, and her ever-constant support system. This is a journey that you can make successfully because, after all, she is worth it.

Resilient

A girl with ADHD, listen closely, please,
To the gentle whisper of self-compassion's ease.

In the swirling storm of thoughts and distraction,
Here's a path to your inner satisfaction.

First, accept your beautiful mind's unique flow,
ADHD's colors in the rainbow you show.

See the strengths it brings, creativity's gift,
Your spirit's uplift, your unique drift.

When focus falters and tasks seem grand,
Remember, self-worth isn't built on shifting sand.

Forgive yourself for moments when you struggle,
In your imperfection, you remain humble.

Acknowledge the wins, no matter how small,
Each step you take, you give your all.

Celebrate your courage to face each day,
With ADHD, you find your own way.

In moments of chaos and overwhelm's embrace,
Step back, breathe deep, find your tranquil space.

Learn to prioritize, break tasks into parts,
You'll find clarity in the midst of the arts.

Seek support and understanding from those who care,
Know you're never alone in this unique affair.

Share your journey, let your voice be heard,
In vulnerability, you'll find your strength stirred.

Be patient, my dear, as you learn and grow,
With love and acceptance, let self-kindness flow.

You're a girl with ADHD, a radiant star,
Embrace your journey for who you truly are.

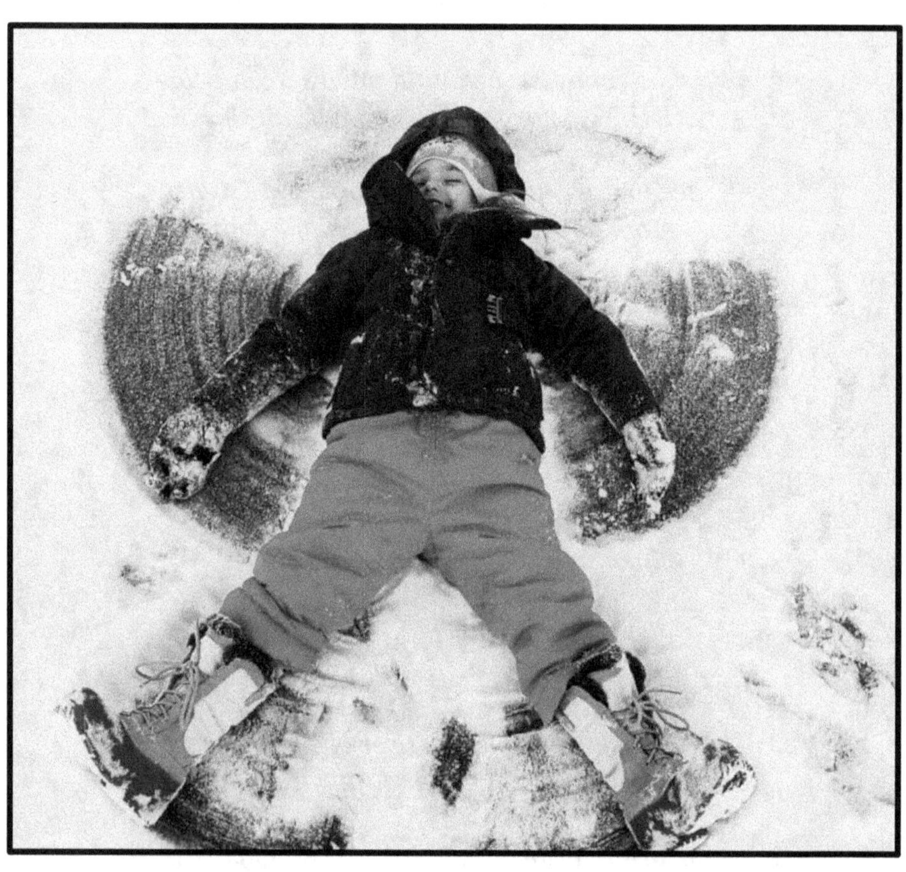